PENGUIN
ARKANA

D0745333

COMA: THE DREAMBOD

A key figure in the field of dream and bodywork, psychological interventions in psychiatry and in conflict resolution, Arnold Mindell is the author of *Dreambody*, *Working with the Dreaming Body*, *River's Way*, *City Shadows*, *Working on Yourself Alone*, *The Year I*, *The Dreambody in Relationships* and with Amy Mindell, *Riding the Horse Backwards* (all published by Arkana). He is an analyst in private practice, co-founder of the Centre for Process Oriented Psychology, Zurich and Portland, and analyst and teacher at these centres. He has been a resident teacher at Esalen Institute, Big Sur, California, and lectures and teaches throughout the world.

ARNOLD MINDELL

COMA: THE DREAMBODY NEAR DEATH

ARKANA

PENGUIN BOOKS

ARKANA

Published by the Penguin Group
Penguin Books Ltd, 27 Wrights Lane, London W8 5TZ, England
Penguin Books USA Inc., 375 Hudson Street, New York, New York 10014, USA
Penguin Books Australia Ltd, Ringwood, Victoria, Australia
Penguin Books Canada Ltd, 10 Alcorn Avenue, Toronto, Ontario, Canada M4V 3B2
Penguin Books (NZ) Ltd, 182- 190 Wairau Road, Auckland 10, New Zealand

Penguin Books Ltd, Registered Offices: Harmondsworth, Middlesex, England

First published by Shambhala Publications, Inc. 1989
Published with a foreword in Penguin Books 1994
3 5 7 9 10 8 6 4 2

To
Ursi Jean

CONTENTS

FOREWORD TO THE ARKANA EDITION

We are happy to see an Arkana edition of *Coma: The Dreambody Near Death* because, since its first Shambhala edition in 1989, we have learned a great deal from working with people from various parts of the world who were near death or re-entering life. Medical personnel and other care givers who came to our seminars to learn about approaching people in deep altered states of consciousness gave us greater confidence in our work.

Our most recent learning can be grouped under two categories: I Structural Comas and II General Theory of Near Death Experiences.

I COMAS FROM STRUCTURAL BRAIN INJURIES

Since the first edition of this work, we have had a lot of experience with people who entered into comatose states from strokes, drug overdose, automobile accidents, near drowning, suffocation due to strangulation and general oxygen deficit, and brain injury resulting from brutal assault.

The work presented in the main text discusses comatose experiences due mainly to metabolic changes near death and is equally applicable to these more traumatic injuries. The difference of course is that, in the case of traumatic injury, the return to normal states of consciousness is slower because the organs of expression have been injured. Nevertheless, we have seen astonishing experiences even when severe brain injury was present where apparently "hopeless" clients, who were hospitalized at the time, roused and expressed themselves in primal ways through groaning and moving.

However, working with people with traumatic brain damage needs greater patience because, though recuperation often happens, it takes weeks or months depending upon the injury. Bodywork with structural damage requires details which are difficult to write about. Some of these can only be learned through "hands-on" training such as touching deep muscles and moving body parts in conjunction with the breath in order to aid body awareness.

Amy has found in her classes that learners are often shy about getting close to or touching people in altered states and sometimes are unnecessarily shy about mirroring and amplifying the primal sounds people make in these states. We can only encourage care givers to attempt to communicate with comatose people in a compassionate and intimate manner, because it reduces their isolation, allows them to express deep things, and facilitates living or dying as the case may be. Hospice workers have often told us that their clients feel better when approached as recommended.

II General Theory

The entire work with people in altered states of consciousness is complex and difficult, not because it is difficult to work with people in these states but because many of us are not at peace with our own death. On the one hand, learning about death and dying is a matter of practice, and on the other it is a matter of personal development or inner work. Fantasies about dying for those of us in normal health often mean learning to let go of aspects of ourselves which are tired and worn out. Our inability to let go and let things happen inhibits life by resisting death. There is a time for this resistance of course, but, if we continue to hang on and form sentimental ties to aspects of life which need dropping, we also hang on to the dying person and make life and death unnecessarily difficult for her or him.

The less centered we are, ourselves, in the processes of life and death, the more we inhibit the client's awareness and communication on these topics. Ill people are often uncomfortable speaking with others who seem against disease, death or permanent injury. The more open and detached we are about such states, the better it is for everyone. But the only way to get there, is to work on ourselves. The method of "practicing your death" and facing the various feelings and unfinished business around your own demise still seems the easiest way to begin in this area.

Buddhism has a great deal to offer here. We have been impressed with the work and teachings of Ondrea and Stephen Levine. Also we want to recommend the work of Sogyal Rinpoche on Tibetan Buddhism. From the teachings of the ancient Tibetans we have developed the viewpoint that many people pass through comatose states into death, while others seems to go in the opposite direction, passing through death-like comatose states, getting stuck coming back to life. In a way, some accident victims are trying to be born again.

At all times, it is most realistic to work with comatose processes assuming that the goal and direction of life are unknown. After all, none of us knows what life is really about. Under these circumstances, we can only follow the nature of the dreaming body experience and its subtle cues, regardless of where these processes may lead us. In this way, life itself remains the teacher.

Amy and Arny Mindell, 1993

PREFACE

Why do I feel a sense of urgency in writing this book? Is it because I am fighting for a new ethics, an extension of the present medical definition of brain death? Or do I need to study near-death experiences in order to discover my own timeless self?

From the beginning, writing this book has been an emotional necessity for me. Even editing this work, months after having written its first draft, I again sense the same urgency that originally inspired me to write. After witnessing the astonishing awakening of Peter from a profound coma, an event described in the first part of this book, I sat down and wrote for days. Some months later my parents died within days of each other. My mother died after having awakened from a coma in the last stages of life, and my father died right after telling me that he wanted to be with her.

I am immensely grateful to Sandy for having asked me to help Peter with his last experiences and for the chance to look at his dreambook, from which portions of this book came. Peter and Sandy inspired me to write this book.

Amy Mindell contributed to every stage of this manuscript, from helping me during the night of Peter's awakening, to helping with the final editing. Thanks also go to Pearl and Carl Mindell, Ursi Jean, Barbara Croci, Dawn Menken, and Nancy Zenoff for valuable suggestions and critical reading. Julie Diamond's editing was immensely helpful.

Various authors have educated me about death and dying. First and foremost, I want to thank Elizabeth Kübler-Ross for having made the study of dying an accepted theme. Without her work and her warm support I would have hesitated even longer to write this book. Thanks to Marie-Louise von

Franz (1986) for her cross-cultural correlation of afterlife theories, which made my dreambody theories more coherent. Sandol Stoddard (1978) exposed the coolness of medical aid and demonstrated humane ways to connect with the dying. Glenn Mullin (1974), Frederick Holck (1978), and others have brilliantly elucidated various insights about death from the Eastern traditions.

Raymond Moody (1976) investigated "out-of-body experiences" occurring near clinical death, laying the foundation for my mythbody concepts. Stephen Levine's (1984) Buddhist meditative practice with dying people is a first stage to dreambody work with comas. Stanislav Grof and Joan Halifax (1978) have amplified death experiences by showing the relationship between LSD and dying. Thanks to them all for having opened the way into a very mysterious territory.

PART ONE

THE KEY TO LIFE

1

A BIG SHIP

This book describes dream work and body work with the dying and methods for unfolding the incomprehensible appearance and unknown purpose of comatose states. I use verbatim bedside reports, theoretical discussions, and practical exercises.

One of my goals is to familiarize the reader with the wide range of unusual events that most of us will encounter near death. Knowing about these events can increase our appreciation of life's end and enrich us by making these altered states a more integral part of our everyday life. Anyone interested in death and dying and other altered states will find hints here for transforming the pain, confusion, and mystery of death into a meaningful experience.

This work questions the belief that comas are unconscious, inaccessible states and that those in persistent vegetative states are—or should be considered—dead. I hope to show that such opinions are unjustified since they are based upon our limited ability to communicate with the comatose state. I describe my work with near-death conditions and the peak experiences to which such work often leads. This work, which uses the methods of process-oriented psychology, makes us interested, optimistic, and even excited about the final stages of life. Process-oriented psychology is a wide-spectrum phenomenological approach to people based upon their verbal and nonverbal signals and states of consciousness. It now seems possible and important to work with comatose states—that is, to work with the often subtle messages they can signal to us—because they contain a veritable treasure of information about life for the dying person and her family.[1] Without amplifying and unfolding, these experiences just leave us baffled and confused in the final and turbulent stages of life.

All those with whom I have worked with while they were comatose have responded readily to the process-oriented communication described in chapter 8. We need to learn a form of communication that appreciates and understands the smallest signals, the most minimal cues of our depths and joys. Once we succeed in communicating with people in strongly altered states, life after death appears as a timeless, eternal reality trying to manifest itself in the present.

Learning how to give the comatose individual access to his or her own depths and communicative abilities should be, I hope, a contribution to a new "Thanatos ethics,"[2] an ethics capable of giving the individual the opportunity to make a clear and conscious choice about life and death, thereby rendering legal debates about life and death obsolete.

PROCESS WORK

My particular approach is based upon process-oriented psychology.[3] Readers interested in the application of dream work and body work near death need not be familiar with process work to follow this book. Wherever possible, I present the ideas and methods from the beginning.

Though work with the dying has been a relatively frequent part of my everyday practice for the past twenty-five years, I have, until now, never written about near-death experiences. Quite honestly, I have hesitated to relate my experiences with the dying due to the work's unusual nature.

A series of events mentioned in this book pressed me to devote my time to this research. I offer it now as a new direction in psychotherapy and in the study of death, rather than as a final statement about the nature of comas. The case material presented here indicates that comatose people are not necessarily in pain; they are not simply brain-damaged vegetables in need of oxygen, suffering from the limbic lobe syndrome triggered by endorphins or like substances. Nor are they merely machines whose central nervous systems, stimulated by extreme physical states, produce haphazard hallucinations and visions. Rather, they are wakeful human beings going through one more meaningful step in their process of individuation.

In fact, people in comas resemble mythical heroes. Storytellers the world over have always enchanted us with tales of the shaman, the king, and the hero, figures who journey through the outermost gates of reality seeking information in the unknown reaches of existence to return with a divine message for the rest of us.

The near-death stupors and comatose states I have worked with often produce symbols of these mythical trips to other worlds. Many of these patients venture to the heights and depths to find some degree of ecstasy, prophetic insight, and self-knowledge.

I did not undertake this study to prove these points, but discovered them en route. Each reader should draw his or her own conclusions from the empirical material. I am not interested in proving or disproving religious or legal views about mortality. Rather, my focus lies in following human nature and helping myself and others to realize who we are, regardless of the implications.

The perennial religious experiences that have been attributed to life after death can certainly be experienced in this life. The dying have helped me to love this world by realizing its unbounded potential for meaning and depth. As a physicist, I was already aware of the theoretical relativity of our world. Now, the application of process work makes theoretical physics look like a dream coming true. Space, time, and locality pale against the colorful involvement of following life to completion.

Peter and Sandy are the fictitious names given to two very real people who are the main figures of this first section.

Peter, a middle-aged man dying of leukemia, experienced fully the dreams, fantasies, symptoms, and relationship issues filling the last days and minutes of his life. The shocking story of awakening that occurred in the final hours of Peter's life gives us the message that we go on growing whether or not time has run out on the physical body.

In the second part of the book, I describe the theory of altered states and give practical hints for the layperson and professional in working with comatose conditions. In the final pages of the book, I wrestle with eternal questions about life, death, and the afterlife.

Sandy's courage, Peter's experiences, and Amy's assistance pushed me past my initial reserve to write about my previous experiences with the dying. Up until recently I had been too shocked, amazed, touched, and dumbfounded by the final processes of life to write about them for fear of doubtful reactions. As far as I knew, sudden awakening from comas had never been written about before. I had only worked alone with dying clients, but now I needed the presence of Amy, Sandy, and Sandy's friend Helen to begin writing.

OUR INTEREST IN DEATH

Why are we now opening up to the experiences in extreme states? As new psychological techniques for awareness arise, many people are becoming dissatisfied with a concept of reality that has no place for visions and ecstatic states. Thus death experiences may hold interest for us because we are seeking to find in them concrete verification for our transpersonal dreams.

Today's public is more interested in caring for its own health and less prepared to give the entire responsibility for life and health to the medical community. While we are thankful for advances in medicine that prolong and enrich life, we are also suspicious of the scientific attitude that approaches the human being as a biomechanical entity whose mental behavior, especially near death, is organized by metabolic and structural pathologies. Yet many still think of themselves as machines, believing that when the machine is irreparably damaged, the human being no longer exists.

Could it also be that public interest in dying indicates that humanity is at a crossroads, a time of transition when old beliefs are dying? Are we now facing a time of reorientation, of seeking a new outlook? If so, looking at death experiences can certainly be of help to us.

Certain cultural taboos still inhibit our interest in dying. For some, death is unmentionable because of the powerful experiences awaiting us there. For others, it is too painful and sad to deal with. And for most of us, regardless of our beliefs, the ever-present threats of loss of our loved ones and confrontation with our own mortality are reasons enough to avoid the topic.

It seems to me, however, that process work has the potential to help us deal with the fear of death and dying because the work is often so relieving. In fact, this work can be not only illuminating but sometimes even fun. Death can be a wonderful time of learning for everyone. The mores and rules of social life diminish in the face of comas and trances, and the pure drive for self-knowledge increases. At death people are prepared more than ever to live fully. Some actually return to life from the depth of apparently terminal comas. Even those who have been opposed to the teachings of psychology and religion become fascinated by their own inner processes near death.

COMAS AND AWAKENINGS

Except for those with severe structural brain damage, all the comatose people I have seen have awakened and verbally communicated powerful experiences. Even those with extensive traumatic brain damage responded positively to process work with nonverbal signals, while those without severe brain damage awakened and completed their unfinished learning and loving. Some died, while others climbed out of bed at the point of death, discharged themselves from the hospital, and went back to life. Most transcended the ideas of life and death altogether, and one person went for a cruise in the Bahamas. Let me tell you his story.

John, a man in this eighties, seemed stuck at the edge of life, unable to die. He had been in and out of semicomatose states for six months, intermittently groaning and yelling. When I saw him he was lying in his hospital bed, moaning and shouting out something that no one could understand. He disturbed the other patients and nurses. Though I was working with a client in another room, the nurses begged me to go in and see him because they thought maybe I could quiet him down.

As I entered his room, I saw an old black man lying in a pool of sweat, groaning loudly. I joked, "Hey! No one around here can get any sleep! You're too loud." John seemed not to hear me but continued to moan.

I decided to follow his sounds. "Ohhh, oooh, wow, yeah," I groaned with him, approximating the sound of his breathing. I gently squeezed his hand in cadence with his respiration and heartbeat.

After about twenty minutes his muffled shouts became distinguishable words. John, who had not said a word to anyone in days or uttered a complete sentence in six months, now said, "Yeah. Wow, No, yeah, . . . oh . . ."

(The following dialogue was recorded on tape)

ARNY (*adding a phrase onto his words*): Wow, yeah, *unbelievable!*

JOHN (*slowly, at first vaguely*): Yeah, you . . . you . . . know . . .

ARNY: Me . . . yeah.

JOHN: Shhhh . . . Yeah. A b . . . bb . . . bbbbiiig, a *biiig* shhhhhip.

ARNY: Shhhhiiiip . . . Yeahhh. Larger than I thought, that ship.

JOHN: Yeah, aaaa *big ship's* . . . coming . . . for John!!!

ARNY: Wow, wow . . . You gonna take it?

JOHN (*yelling with all his might*): No, man—*not me!!* I'm not getting on that ship.

ARNY: Why not?

JOHN (*long pause, coughing and sputtering*): That ship's goin'
. . . on . . . vacation! I'm not going. I gotta get up at eight in
the morning and go to work!

ARNY: Me too. Me too . . . But do me a favor, a big favor
(*following the direction of John's eye motions*), put your eyes
up in your head and take a good look at the ship.

(John began to look incredulous and rolled his head upwards.)

ARNY: Look in and then tell me who's driving that ship.

JOHN: Hummm, who . . . hmmm. (*Looking up, the whites of his
eyes showing*) Oh wow!! Wow . . . There are angels in that
ship, driving it.

ARNY: Angels?

I feel excited and think to myself that this experience has to
be completed, that is, he has to go into it more deeply in
order for it to be of use to him.

ARNY: Take a look in the boiler room. Who's in there?

JOHN (*looking down, moving his head down*): Hmmmm. Oh
wow, hmmm, down there . . . angels . . . too. No . . . Yeah.
(*Though limited by his physical deterioration, he begins to
yell with excitement*) Hey . . . Heyyy . . . Heeey . . . Angels
are driving that ship!!

ARNY: *Angels! Woww!* Please do me a favor, will ya? Go closer
and check out just how much it costs to get on that ship.

JOHN: Hmm . . . (*looking from side to side*) hmm, yeah, yeah.
That . . . no . . . yeah . . . that . . . well . . . it costs nothing.
Ze . . . ro.

ARNY: Well, what do you think about that? It's a free trip.

JOHN: Interesting. Yeah!

ARNY: You ever had a vacation?

JOHN: Nope, not me.

ARNY: Listen man, you never had a vacation. You're a working
man. You should consider a little trip. If you don't like it, you
can come back. If you like it, then think it over. If you want
to, take off. Come back if you want or just keep going. You
can now make all the decisions yourself. If you go on vacation
and stay, good. If you stay here, fine. If you go, I'd love to
meet you there some day.

JOHN: Yeah. Yeah. Vacation, to the Bahamas, Ba . . . ha . . .
mas . . . Yeah. Hmmmm . . . no work.

John quieted down, closed his eyes and went to sleep. He
had stopped screaming. I went back to my client and came

back about half an hour later to see what he was up to. A nurse was standing by his bed and said that John had just died. I was both sad and happy. The old man had decided to go on vacation.

Though I would have loved to have known him better, at least I had the chance to help him relax his work ethic and take a trip to the Bahamas. He needed a break from working. He was stuck at the edge of life because he was in conflict about whether or not he could go on vacation. He was also stuck because those around him had trouble communicating with the yelling and hooting of his comatose state.

For John, his coma state may have been a statement like this: "I am in conflict. There is no one here who can help me with it, so I'll do the best I can by going internal and visualizing this ship. Since I am not used to working with visions, I can only shout with excitement about what I see."

Today, as never before, the needs of the dying are being met in hospices, hospitals, and private homes with loving-kindness, psychological understanding, silent meditation, and prayer. Yet some of the deepest inner feelings of the dying—like John's conflict about vacation—escape our attention. All of us connected with the dying do the best we can, but we are still in the beginning stages of our work. There is still a lot to learn about dying, as we can see by the frustration we feel in our inability to relate to the dying. We guess incorrectly that they are unreachable, that they are leaving their bodies, and that compassion, meditation, and love are all we can offer. All of these interventions are necessary, but none are sufficient.

Most dying people need assistance to experience fully the powerful events trying to happen. Without assistance, altered states confuse and baffle us. We misinterpret the signals of an altered state, believing they are signs of pain, drugs, or disease. While the dying silently and alone seek the solutions to life, we misunderstand them and imagine that they are peacefully floating off to another world.

2

CROSSING THE BRIDGE

Psychotherapeutic work with a patient in the early stages of a severe illness does not essentially differ from work in other stages of life. The gravity of death, however, gives the work greater intensity. In the early stages of severe illness, the client's goals usually aim at healing the problem. Some who come to me become interested in discovering the experiences manifested in the symptoms. Integrating this psychology frequently reduces the gravity of the symptoms. Thus the early work is characterized by a conflict between the present conscious behavior and new aspects of the personality that emerge in dreams and symptoms.[1] I have often found that people who had previously been unable to make large changes, suddenly, in their last moments, took quantum jumps toward their totality.

Let us now meet Peter and Sandy and consider some of the details of working with Peter during the last three weeks of his life.

PETER

I was on vacation around the turn of the year, trying to escape from the turmoil of city life by retreating to the Alps. A telephone call broke through the quiet of a dark Alpine evening. The distressed voice on the other end said, ''One of my relatives is dying of leukemia, and we would like your help! We have been told that he has one or two days to live."

The caller was Peter's sister-in-law. I replied that if Peter really wanted to live and to work with us, and if this were really the right thing to do, nature would help him wait until we were able to meet him in the hospital. Two weeks later we met for the first time at a hospital in Zurich. Peter, his wife, Sandy, and my wife, Amy, were present. Amy had agreed to help me with the relationship work and with the emotional load that we felt could occur.

Before we entered the hospital room, Sandy told us that Peter had never had any interest in psychology. He disliked religion. It had only been since his last near-fatal leukemia crisis that he had even shown any interest in speaking about his feelings. As we entered, I was happy to find Peter in an apparently good mood, lying quietly in bed, moving his legs occasionally in response to our conversation. An introverted, highly intelligent middle-aged man, he looked physically reduced and ashen.

After the introductions were over, I asked Peter what, if anything, he would still like to accomplish in his life. I was looking for that special spot, that growing edge, where we all work. I wondered if he could identify such a spot. This spot is the edge (see Glossary), a place where we get stuck and cannot go further. At the edge of our development we turn around and become sick, become unconscious, or go crazy. It is the point which we cannot get by, the spot where we get depressed and hopeless.

Peter answered immediately that if he could, he would put his relationship with Sandy in order. They had been emotionally disconnected for some time. I speculated with Sandy and Peter at the end of our introductory session that one of our jobs would be to work on their marriage. I recommended that in spite of his weakened body condition we do some form of relationship work together. I suggested that I see Peter alone first in the hospital before we all met together again as a foursome, and asked Sandy to see Amy in the meantime. I felt that my main task would be to focus on his inner process and his illness; the second job would be to process their relationship issues and discover how they connected, if at all, to his symptoms. Amy and I hoped that by working together and separately with them, their individual changes would allow them to transform as a couple.

THE HOME SITUATION

Sandy appeared to be a highly intelligent, courageous, and creative woman who was willing to try anything that might help her family and herself. Amy reported about her work with Sandy,

> When I arrived at their home, I played with the kids while Sandy was busy with the incredible number of domestic tasks connected to balancing a household with the hospital visits. Their apartment was orderly, colorful, with a lot of children's pictures and toys around. There were also many books and records lying about, giving the impression of a family with many interests.
>
> The eldest child was very excited about his new train set. Sandy told the kids to speak slowly because my Swiss German was not so good. The eldest became interested in my cheap watch. He thought I was rich and hid my watch in another room. He and the middle child started to fight playfully with me until Sandy came in. She was upset because the kids had messed up some of the clothes folded on the bed. The eldest told me that the devil slept under his bed. I thought to myself that changes in this family might well happen in the direction of less order and more devilishness.

Amy told me that Sandy spoke of how difficult life had become since Peter's illness. She was both sad and angry at Peter for not having gone into therapy earlier. She said that when they fought Peter would withdraw into his room, play the guitar, and then come out and talk quietly about their problems. It seemed that they were both a bit shy about emotional expression. Sandy said that the eldest boy's temperament sometimes clashed with hers. The youngest, she said, sat at the head of the dinner table and slept in a crib in their bedroom. It appeared that the identified family process was to be loving, while wild or sensitive emotions or expressions of feeling were waiting under the surface to be expressed.

When Amy asked Sandy what sort of things she wanted in life, she replied, like Peter, that she wanted to work out their relationship issues and get to the love that she felt was there. She talked glowingly and lovingly of him, and showed Amy pictures of him playing with the children. She said that she could never be as sensitive and playful as he could be. It was a very good sign that both she and Peter shared the goal of working on their relationship.

Amy reported that after the third session, when Peter began to come out with his need for greater sensitivity, Sandy got depressed because she had never learned how to express her most sensitive feelings. She seemed shy about going into those feelings. In fact it was not her way, at that time, to act out her sensitive feelings. She was apparently determined to use her strength. Amy encouraged her to use her strength to connect to her courage. She used it to express her own ideas to the medical team about how she would like Peter to be treated. She needed to fight, rather than feel, at that point.

First Session with Peter

In my first session alone with Peter, I told him to feel free to tell me everything about himself that he felt was important. When he said he did not dream, I told him that I needed his dreams to check out if we were on the right track, as I did not trust my own suggestions. I said that I hoped he would have a dream that night to help us both. In the days that followed, Peter became a prolific dreamer.

He was very interested in telling me about himself and said that he was a man who could easily fall in love. The women he had met until now tended to be very shy about relationships. He said that he needed a more sensitive and delicate feeling contact with Sandy, and that if this did not happen, he would consider separation.

I told him that a lot of dying people I had met used their death as a means of separating from difficult situations, and that there might be other ways of solving relationship problems. As our first session came to an end, I praised him for speaking so openly and challenged him to tell Sandy about some of his feeling needs, even though it had not been customary for them to talk so directly in the past.

That night when Sandy came to the hospital he told her about his wish for more sensitivity and romance. He later told me that she had become angry and then depressed because he had never said such things earlier. I imagined that she must have become irritated because he probably used his unfulfilled needs as a weapon to make her feel guilty for not fulfilling them. Peter said that Sandy had countered his requests by saying that she thought all of this might be too late; she was not certain she knew how to give him what he wanted. This interaction set off a series of dreams that he told me about during our second session.

FIRST DREAMS

In Peter's diary, I read that

> contact with Arny has unblocked me. My dreams fascinate me now and give me positive support for my will to live.

Then he reported the following dream to me:

> I am climbing up the supporting column of a bridge. The winds are blowing wildly (he moves his arms like a vibrating column back and forth while explaining this part of the dream) and have ripped the bridge up a bit. Engineers and workers are trying to piece it back together again. I manage to climb from the river below up to the surface of the bridge. I cross the bridge and find myself sitting safely on the other side.

He drew a picture of this dream, showing himself on the other side of a ravine, and then a bridge being hastily put back together again.

Peter took to therapy like a fish to water. As soon as he had told me the dream, he wanted to know everything about it and also about his body experiences. He asked me why his legs were twitching so much. At that point, I was shy for some reason to do body work with him and focused on his interest in the dream. I explained to him that the body experiences could wait; we would probably find the same information in his dreams.

I asked him what came to mind in connection with the destruction of a bridge. He told me that the Swiss army did not allow soldiers to march in step (*Gleichschritt*) because the rhythm could set off the bridge's natural vibrating frequency and cause it to shake to pieces. He also said that sometimes great winds and storms could ruin a bridge. Speaking of the army prompted him to say that he always had a tendency to behave in a very standard way. He was a "solid citizen." He would go home every evening after work, get up early every morning, be decent, well-meaning, and constant in his life tempo. He had a militarylike inner discipline.

I said to him that his regularity might also disturb the ability to make changes and to move on to new things. He laughed and admitted that this was true. He had always been too much of a regular guy.

I mentioned how death had always been imagined as a bridge to the beyond, to the other world. The other world was, I guessed, the place where one could live everything that was impossible in this life. Peter excitedly agreed with this. "I must already be on the other side," he said, "for I never would have believed that I could have told Sandy last night about my most intimate feelings!"

"Congratulations," I said. "You crossed your first bridge."

BODY WORK

I asked Peter how he knew he had leukemia. He said that he could not feel it directly in his body. His only symptom was fatigue. He complained of a slight tremor, which he attributed to an attack of flu. As he told me about the shaking, he shook his arms in the same way he had done when telling me about the winds blowing the bridge. I encouraged him to continue shaking, and he shook with conviction for some minutes. Suddenly he stopped and asked if he could be shaking with fear. Fear of what? I asked. Fear of dying and of the new emotions coming up that he had not known before, he said. He was afraid of his needs, his rage and fear. Yet even though he was afraid, he wanted to develop his feelings further. I promised him I would help him to bridge the change and weather the storm. Then he asked me how.

> ARNY: Shake some more now.
> PETER (*involuntarily shaking*): Oh, I am a bit shaky.
> ARNY: And?
> PETER: Will I die?
> ARNY (*jokingly*): Peter, I guarantee that you shall die. Why wait? How about dying now?
> PETER: What?
> ARNY: Pretend you are dying. Just pretend.
> PETER: OK.

Peter stopped shaking, closed his eyes and seemed to rest. After a moment, he opened them again and spoke to me.

> PETER: Something has stopped. I am in touch with peace. I feel so close to you.

He shyly reached out one hand to me and we held hands.

> ARNY (*softly*): Congratulations, you have crossed the bridge again, this time to your feelings. It was scary, but you did it. The beyond must be here now.
> PETER: I love it.

A FAMILY SESSION

Several days later we had a second family meeting. Amy and I were both there. Peter lay in the hospital bed, and Sandy sat in a chair nearby. Sandy and Peter spoke about each other while facing me. I asked Peter to notice the difference between facing me, as he was doing, and facing Sandy. After turning hesitantly to her, he said that if their problems did not clear up, he wanted a separation. I asked if the significance of his facing me and not her was an indirect way to avoid making such a strong statement.

Before he could answer, Sandy reacted by looking down at the floor. She began to play with her shoelaces. She shyly examined her fingernails. I went over to her, took her hand in mine, and said that I liked how she looked at her nails.

She replied that she had always bitten them as a child. I asked her how old she was when she had bitten her nails. Twelve, she said.

"Why not try being a twelve-year-old now?" I recommended, hoping that her somatic reactions to Peter's threat of separation would come to awareness.

She cocked her head to one side and smiled coquettishly. Peter smiled lovingly and said, "That is exactly why I am in love with you." Sandy became angry and said she did not want to be identified only as a child.

"Good," I said. "Being a child and begging for love is not the person you want to be in dealing with his ultimatum. What is your way of dealing with this situation? How would you like to react, and how would you like to be identified?"

"As a woman with a mind and heart of her own!" Sandy replied.

"Good," I said, "and how does that woman react to Peter?" Sandy began to cry, and said she was hurt. We were all quiet for a moment and felt sad about the conflict between them.

She next countered his ultimatum by saying that she did not like his hobby of buying fast cars because it was not good for the environment. When he didn't reply, something seemed to change in her. Her voice dropped and she confided to him how meaningful his needs really were to her. She said she appreciated his interests now. Both came very close to their feelings as the session ended.

Peter had apparently been shy about facing Sandy with his unhappiness. When he went over his edge of shyness and threatened her, she hesitated, then went over an edge, and became angry and hurt. These emotional processes connected them, as they crossed the first of many feeling bridges to come.

Mythologically, the bridge over the river is the road to heaven that transcends both earth and death. Peter's trembling bridge symbolizes the terrifying passage from his known self to unknown feelings and contact, to a "heaven on earth." The bridge is man-made and thus a conscious construction, one we all need to make between different states of consciousness. This myth is for us all. We are all in danger of either stopping at the brink of new behavior or of falling into the river and floating unconsciously in the stream of events. The bridge represents our potential for transcending the unconscious stream of life and connecting to more expressive and rich behavior.

3

THE DEATH
SENTENCE

Peter called me at my practice from the hospital. He had a good reason. In a depressed voice he told me that the doctor and his hospital residents had come to his room to inform him that his leukemia was not responding to the treatment, and that they expected he would die shortly. They recommended that he tell his family to come to say good-bye. The residents had been coming in every half hour and repeating the message.

On the phone Peter cried and said that what he needed was not a death sentence, but support to keep on living. I encouraged him to tell the doctor his feelings, and to ask him to stop the assistants from repeating the message.

I called the hospital and explained to the doctor that I understood it was important to inform a patient that his disease was no longer responding to treatment and that he could die. But, I added, the staff should realize that the way they inform their patient has the effect of a hypnotic induction and could be murderous. There are many ways to tell a patient that the treatment is not successful and that the prognosis is poor. But to tell a patient "You will die soon" is a form of murder.

The doctor argued that directness was the best way. He proceeded to tell me how badly he felt that he could no longer help. He admitted to being angry with Peter for dying. The doctor wanted him to live but felt helpless. I said that all those feelings, not just some of them, would certainly be useful for Peter to hear. We concluded in mutual understanding.

But this "death sentence," as Peter called it, had already had a demoralizing effect. Peter's mood got progressively worse with each visit from a doctor. He began to fantasize about leaving the hospital. I supported his desires, hoping to get him to a clinic with a warmer atmosphere or even to bring him home. But we did not have time.

LOVE DREAMS

His dreams transcended all of our plans. When I called him on the phone the next day, he reported the following dream:

> I am in bed with Sandy and another woman. The other woman is shy. I too am very shy. She is someone I could fall in love with.

We decided to work together on the phone.

PETER: I can see this woman clearly.
ARNY: Peter, why don't you visualize her as completely as possible?
PETER: Hmm, very pretty.
ARNY: Yes, I can almost see her. Isn't she good-looking? What color is her hair?
PETER: Brown. She sounds so warm.

I noticed that he switched from visualizing her to hearing her voice. I went along and switched channels (see Glossary) with him.

ARNY: Her voice is pleasant. What is her name?
PETER: It could be French. She is erotic and lovely.
ARNY: Sounds like a good dream! What's it like to be in bed with two women at once, one of whom is French?
PETER: Very supportive, very loving. I love Sandy, too.

I thought that the French woman was symbolic of his feelings, but hoped he would discover this himself.

ARNY: What is it really like in bed? I am not quite there with you yet.

PETER: The French woman has brown hair. Is she a woman from work? No, that woman is too shy and would not even visit me in the hospital. I see a dark-haired woman, thin, bright, but not too intelligent because feeling is so important.
ARNY: Go on, fantasize about her.

Peter began to have an inner dialogue with this French woman. She was a very feeling, emotional, and high-spirited woman. As he continued the imagination, he discovered that she had a fighting spirit, a capacity to fight for life. Spontaneously, he added that Sandy, too, had that fighter's spirit.

ARNY: In your dream, you and Sandy are together in part because you share this French personality, this feeling about life. It is a feeling of warmth, support, and the desire to fight for life.

Peter, who had been depressed until this point, enthusiastically agreed. We talked a bit more, and then I told him, "Shut your eyes and get into bed with those women now." I did not see him on the other end of the phone, but heard him sighing contentedly. "Thank you," he said.

DREAM WORK

I came to the hospital at lunchtime the next day. Peter's physical condition had deteriorated. He greeted me and without waiting told me the following dream.

I am in bed with an unknown woman. A second woman who has been sleeping nearby also wants to get into bed with us but is too shy.
Two men are playing with fire nearby. I tell them not to be too wild with the fire. Then I see a sleeping woman lying at the base of my bed and I pick her up so she will not have to be on the floor. She asked me why I awakened. "I had to," I said.

Apparently this dream had picked up from where we left off. He was again with the shy, unknown woman. I wondered to myself what events in his life he still experienced as shy and unknown.

> ARNY: Who are the men? If you were to play with fire, what would you do?
> PETER: I would stop taking medication and leave the hospital. I would go out and have a good time.

I was in a rush and couldn't stay long. Just as I was leaving, Peter asked me what the dream meant. I tried to get him to tell me what he thought it meant, but he persisted and wanted to know what I thought. Assuming that dreams are processes trying to happen in consciousness, I told him not to be surprised if he soon forgot the conflict with the hospital scene, became detached from the life-and-death dilemma, and "burned." I told him to "burn a little." He then changed the subject.

> PETER: Who was the woman on the floor?
> ARNY: Do you feel "dropped" like she does in some way?
> PETER: It seems that she is someone who has just become hopeless and who needs to be reawakened. I have been hopeless and have almost given up on life.
> ARNY: What would awakening her mean?
> PETER: God only knows. What do you think?
> ARNY: For me there is no life or death anymore, there is only the process of becoming yourself.
> PETER (laughing): You are unbelievable. That would be a real awakening!

We were quiet a few minutes and then I heard him humming something under his breath.

> ARNY: What is the name of that song?
> PETER: Just a little French melody about freedom.
> ARNY: Isn't it great to be freed, to burn off all that we do not need? It's freeing to center on just what is important.
> PETER: Yes, like love.

There are many ways of looking at dreams. Rather than enter into a theoretical discussion about them, I prefer to stay close to what happened. It is useful to understand dreams as descriptions of processes that are only partially in our awareness, processes that are trying to happen with more consciousness. In other words, Peter's dreams implied that a part of him had "dropped out" of the outer situation. Indeed, he was about to enter a coma, drop out of consensus reality, and awaken to a new life.

At the time, however, I assumed that the sleeping woman was a part of him needing to be awakened, perhaps a feeling part that he had "dropped" in some way. I realize only now as I write his story down that the sleeping woman was a symbolic formulation of a powerful experience that was about to happen. He was about to sleep. He needed to drop everything, to enter a coma before he could wake up.

WATERFALLS

I saw Peter again the next day. There was a large assemblage of family and relatives inside and outside his room. Despite the large gathering of relatives, his fever, and his advancing pneumonia, Peter excitedly told me that he had not been able to sleep all night. He asked all his relatives but Sandy to leave while he told me the following dreams.

> I go up into wild waterfalls and come down into a warm and silent pool of water in the midst of a forest. I go up and come down the falls many times.

With barely a breath's pause, he rapidly told me the next dream:

> I am about to get married. A helicopter lands on the ground and a commander comes out. He goes out on the sea with a little rowboat that almost overturns, yet he manages to come back to dry land safely.

I wondered to myself why he was speaking so quickly, what his rush was. Was this the burning from the earlier dream? Was it due to his fever, or was it the excitement of leaving an old consciousness behind? Perhaps his speediness was his irritation with the visitors.

Since Peter had said that he was seeing the waterfalls, I stayed with the visual mode of perceiving and recommended that he see himself going up into the waterfalls. He closed his eyes and a few minutes later told me that he felt the falls. I encouraged him to feel the falls. After a moment's meditation he said without hesitation that the wild water was his fear of dying. I recommended that he ride the falls, that he go into them and shake. I told him to go ahead and be afraid. He began to shake in bed, alternating between a panicky state and a relaxed, sleepy one. After a few moments he came back and said that now he had come down into quiet waters.

"Riding my fear of death is like being in a waterfall," he explained. "It is the natural way to quietness. Uh-oh. Here comes fear again." His eyes seemed terrified and he looked wildly around the room, like a wild animal in danger.

"Ride the wild waters as if it were a natural way," I said to him. He went into his fear as he had done in his dream until he found himself again in silent waters. We both relaxed and were quiet.

He then wanted to meditate. I followed his request, and we both meditated for a while. Then he fell asleep—for the first time in sixty hours, as a nurse informed me. Apparently the fever, shaking, and sleeplessness had been connected with his fear of dying. When he awoke several hours later, his fever had gone down and he felt better.

Riding the sensations of panic had a calming effect on Peter. His dream was apparently showing him how to ride the stream of events. Like the helicopter pilot in his dream, going out to sea and almost drowning, and as in the dream of riding the waterfalls, he was learning how to follow the flow of fear and panic and find his way back to safety and centeredness again.

As I left Peter's room, I was aware of the tense mood prevailing over the group of relatives waiting outside. One relative furiously claimed that Peter should have believed in God earlier. In response, another said that Peter had always been a good boy. Each was dealing with his death in the way he or she knew best. Some of these people had not seen each other for a long time, and they seemed to be using the occasion to work out their family affairs. This also should have been part of my work, but I was too exhausted to help and left Amy and Sandy to deal with the situation.

The next day Peter had trouble breathing and was wearing an oxygen mask. He was in a sleepy state. The nurse told me that his pulse was 150. He was sweating profusely and was not able or willing to communicate.

I held his hand and sang softly. He started moving his legs around in what seemed to be a violent motion for his condition. I gently inhibited the motion of one of his legs in order to amplify the impulse behind its movement. I told him that his legs had the strength to do what he wanted.

Suddenly he sat up, kicked violently, and yelled out loud.

PETER: *Shit!*
ARNY: Shit what? (*yelling*) Say the rest of the sentence!
PETER: Shit that I'm so sick. *Shit Leukemia!*

He was furious with fate. His fever and high pulse were expressions of that rage. After yelling he breathed more freely and pulled off his oxygen mask in a commanding way. He measured his own pulse and said, "I feel better." I said that he looked like a bad boy who had just said a naughty word. "You should always be nice and accept everything that happens to you," I joked. He grinned mischievously.

Just then one of his relatives came in. Peter suddenly gasped for breath, put the mask back on, and fell back down. I asked the relative to wait outside, and gently reprimanded Peter for feigning sleep instead of letting out his angry feelings then and there.

He countered my scolding by saying, "You've got some nerve! You're fresh!" I congratulated him for scolding me back. I said, "It's true. I do have nerve. I say 'shit' when I need to." We both laughed heartily. We admired each other's spunkiness and reveled in the breakthrough. When the next relative came in, Peter told him to leave, laughed, and then fell asleep.

SANDY AND PETER

The next day, I was sitting by Peter as he was sleeping. Sandy came in. She sat next to him and wept.

ARNY: Why are you crying?
SANDY: I now realize how much I've really loved him. I feel that I can't get on alone afterward without him. I'd like to die now, with the kids. I don't want to lose him.

Peter awoke at this point. He looked at her and then looked away. I asked him what he had seen.

PETER: I see that I also love her. Because of that I want to get well.

That was the first time that he had said that he loved her and wanted to live for her. I was very touched. They began to hug each other intimately. I got embarrassed and got up to leave. They asked me to stay.

Later, standing outside with Sandy, she told me that she regretted that Peter was only now learning to love and express feelings. She felt that it was so late. As she spoke of her fear of having to bring up the kids alone, she started to cry. I stayed with her a few more moments and comforted her.

I told her that if she felt like dying, she should do it now in a fantasy. Dying in a fantasy is a way of regenerating. Sandy closed her eyes and I left her with Amy.

The next evening Sandy called and asked over and over again if Peter would die. She wanted to know how I personally felt about death. I avoided the question and said that all I could be certain of was that he was going to change. I had seen many people at this point of dying. Many die, I told her, but others have gotten better, gotten out of bed, and gone back to work.

Because of my having seen so many people die, life and death have a new meaning for me. They are relative concepts. Death is frightening only as long as we identify ourselves with who we have been in life. That is why I recommend to people who worry about death to go through the death fantasy in detail. The fantasy of dying is often the need to drop an attitude or identity that has run out of time. When people imagine that they are dying, they frequently close their eyes, take a pause from their momentary identity, and enter a new phase of life.

I told Sandy that I saw our job as following his and her processes as well as we could and helping them experience consciously whatever was happening. Nature, I trusted, would do the rest. She asked me why I didn't get depressed in hospitals. I replied that my experiences with people led me to believe in nature, because whatever happened always seemed to bring people more than they had even asked for. Death is guaranteed. We have to die, again and again, as new things begin.

Sandy brought me out of my revelations. "What should I do now?" she asked. "Doubt, continue questioning, and call us," I answered.

4

COMA AND REBIRTH

The last night of Peter's life was amazing. It was reminiscent of the dramatic peak religious experiences people have during ordinary life. Yet there was a difference. For Peter, it was an awesome awakening to the secrets of life.

Our last night with Peter began at about eight one evening when Amy called from the hospital. She had gone to visit Peter and found a new doctor standing outside the door of his room. He told her that Peter was dying and no one could enter. Amy called to Sandy who was inside, and Sandy let her in.

COMATOSE STATE

When I arrived, Peter had on the oxygen mask. He was comatose, was breathing heavily and noisily, and was unable to be aroused by usual methods of communication. His hands were grayish blue, and his breathing "rattled" because his lungs were filled with water from the pneumonia. His kidneys had failed, and his body was swollen. He had stopped urinating some hours earlier. He lay motionless in the bed, while the nurses came in periodically, checking technical details. Sandy, her friend Helen, and Amy huddled together, caring for one another. Peter had received some morphine and was scheduled for another dose in several hours.

I sat down on his bed and turned my sad feelings for him into an intense focus upon his process. I looked at his body, listened to his breathing, felt his chest, and searched for the strongest signal. His rasping and irregular breathing were clearly his main signals to the outside world.

Though I understood his irregular and noisy breathing as a result of his disturbed physical condition, I listened to the irregular inhalation and exhalation as his only possible form of communication. I put my hands in his, gently pressing and then releasing my touch in the rhythm of his breathing to experience and feel where he was. Sandy put Peter's favorite music into the cassette player and told me that he loved Mendelssohn's Octet because it was wild and reminded him of her.

I softly spoke to him in the cadence of his breathing. To understand his response to me, I counted his rate of inhalation and exhalation, closely watched the movements of one of his eyebrows, listened to sounds coming from his lungs, and kept track of the color changes in his cheeks and lips. As I spoke to him, I put my lips close to his ear and tracked his reactions. I whispered, in the rhythm of his breathing, something like the following.

"Hello, Peter. This is me, Arny. I am with you again. I am going to hold your hand, and am about to put my hand on your chest. I would like you to believe, as you have in the past, in what is happening to you. Whatever is happening, whatever it is, will show us the way. It is going to be our guide. So continue to feel, see, hear, and move with the feelings, visions, sounds, and movements happening within you. Yes, that's it. This will bring us to wherever we have to go."

As I spoke, Peter remained motionless except for the rasping, irregular breathing and slight eyebrow movements that appeared in connection with my statements. Sandy slept. Amy and I talked, and we intermittently took turns communicating with Peter. The atmosphere in the room filled with a growing awesomeness, the sound of the rasping breath, and a feeling of respect for the unknown.

As the time approached for his next morphine injection, I woke Sandy and recommended that she request that it not be administered. She asked the doctor not to give Peter any more painkillers. The physician insisted that giving him morphine was the most merciful thing to do. He said that he had been through all of this recently with a close relative who had not received enough pain medication and thus suffered a miserable death.

I intervened and said that I believed he had been humane with his relative but that Peter was not in pain. I tried to explain, though in vain, that I knew Peter wasn't in pain because I had been "communicating" with him through the minimal, nonverbal responses to my questions.[1] I was ineffective. I was tired and groggy and could not get my idea across. Just as anyone else in a position of great responsibility might have done, the doctor and medical aides seemed simply to refuse to consider the possibility of a completely new way of thinking in the middle of the night. He remained firm in his decision to administer the morphine injection.

It was then that I thought to myself that I would write a book about nonchemical ways of working with pain. I decided to make it known that there are methods for working with pain that do not cloud consciousness. If these methods do not work, then painkillers may be the best solution. But awareness is the first option, because the individual himself or herself can determine what should happen.

Since that night I have learned to have more compassion with those rendering medical assistance to the dying. Medical professionals are trained to circumvent pain and death as much as possible. Most have not had sufficient opportunity to study the dimensions and processes around pain and the meaningfulness of death, even as a concept.

Sandy insisted that the doctor not administer morphine. The doctor agreed to wait half an hour longer before giving Peter the injection. The conflict with the doctor made the atmosphere tense and difficult to work in.

I reported my conflict with the doctor in a whisper to Peter. I could not detect any noticeable feedback from him, so I assumed that my problems were not his at the moment.

But the next time the doctor came in, Peter himself convinced him that he was not in pain. What happened was the following:

Around 3:30 in the morning, I got tired and wanted to go home for a few hours of sleep. Amy did not agree. She said she could not explain why, but she felt we should remain. I decided to ask Peter what to do. Still talking in the rhythm of his breathing, I quietly and slowly said to him that if he wanted us to stay, he would have to give us stronger signals. I said that the tiny eyebrow signals and skin color changes were insufficient signals to convince me to stay. Without a stronger signal, I would have to go home and go to sleep. I would see him tomorrow.

RESURRECTION

Shocking us all, Peter suddenly sat straight up! Without the help of anyone, Peter left his comatose position, bolted up, turned his head toward me, blinked, and then turned his whole torso to where I was sitting. He focused his eyes on me for a moment, leaned toward me, and then lowered himself gently down again to the bed.

I was in shock. I managed to say weakly, "Hi there," and then I started shaking. Amy and Sandy almost fell out of their chairs in fright. As I regained my composure, I blurted out, "OK, OK, I promise. I'm not going. I'll stay the rest of the night. I'm not tired anymore!"

When the nurses came in, we told them the story. One nurse stood around with us for hours watching what followed. Doctors came by, looked in, and left again. Peter bolted up once again. He intended to live and communicate. He inspired our fatigue away. By sitting up, he had "told" us that he wanted us to stay. Apparently he had more to do.

Shortly thereafter Peter began to come out of his coma. He started to move his lips, and Sandy, now fully awake, wet them with a damp cloth. He looked up at her. We had been making sounds to amplify the noises in his lungs, and now Peter began to make new noises in "answer" to ours. He met our noises with similar ones, and to our surprise, his sounds turned out to be a song-game! He moved his arms to the rhythm of our musical cacophony and then, of all things, he directed us! He pretended to be conducting an orchestra!

Peter, Sandy, Amy, and I continued groaning, moaning and singing. It must have been 5:00 A.M. by then. Our party became so loud that we thought we might disturb the other patients. Luckily, no one bothered us anymore. We were all happy to be able to be with one another in this new and unexpected way.

It is difficult to give the reader the sense we shared of time passing. The events that occurred that night between Peter, Sandy, and the rest of us were enveloped by a sense of mystery, so that hours condensed into minutes. As day broke, we found ourselves in the midst of an ecstatic celebration of life. Our singing had transformed the tense and cold atmosphere surrounding his death into a festival, a kind of welcome-home party.

Peter could now move his arms, and he lovingly embraced Sandy. They both cried and declared their love for each other. It was such a strong and moving gesture that the rest of us cried too. I asked if we should go, but both Sandy and Peter begged us to stay.

VISION

Peter now wandered between wakeful and sleepy states. At one point he gurgled and then sputtered out the following vision.

PETER: 9. That is the number. 9.

ARNY: 9. That's great. 9, 99, 999.

PETER (*excitedly*): Arny, I have found it. *It. I . . . have . . . found . . . the thing . . . I . . . have . . . always . . . looked . . . for . . . the . . . key . . . to . . . life . . . the key . . .*

ARNY: Great. I wondered what you were doing there in bed. Don't hesitate to tell about that key. We all need it.

PETER: The key is . . . No . . . The old plan, yes, the new plan, the key is . . . the new tram plan, the tram lines in Zurich.

ARNY: I love tram plans. They are important. If only I knew more about them.

PETER: Amy and Helen, the two women are in the new plan . . . Wow, yeah. Wow. They are tram stops.

We all stood around his bed, yelling excitedly and following his idea with enthusiasm.

PETER: And also the key is w-o-z-i-e. The number 9.

ARNY: 9. That's great. 9, 99.

PETER: Arny, I have found it. *It. I . . . have . . . found . . . the thing . . . I . . . have . . . always . . . looked . . . for . . . the . . . key . . . to . . . life . . . the key . . .*

ARNY: Great, man. You got the key.

PETER: Yeah! Now I have found it. *W-o-z-i-e.*

We all repeated the word together with him, encouraging him to continue.

ARNY: Great word. Great tram plan.

PETER: Everything is in the plan. Everything.

ARNY: What is in that plan? What does it mean?

PETER: Hmm, hmm. What does it mean?

He stopped singing and echoed my question. I realized that cognitive questions were the wrong track.

ARNY: How foolish of me. Let's sing "wozie."

PETER: Wozie was here even before you began to work with me.

Now we were standing around Peter's bed in a state of excitement and curiosity.

At this point Peter went to sleep, and Amy and I took a break and went down to the cafeteria for breakfast. We began to theorize furiously. What could be the meaning of this "wozie"? *Wo* is German for "where," and "zie" sounds like *sie*, which means "she." Was he saying "where is she?" Was he saying something about the feminine, his feelings? Or could it be that he was saying "what she wants," because "wozie" was also close to the phrase *wott sie* ("she wants") in the Swiss German dialect.

Amy remembered that Peter told us that "wozie" was the original pattern that had been there before we came. Furthermore, "wozie" was prefaced by the number 9 and is also connected in some way to the new Zurich tram plan. Why was all of this communicated to us as a loving and festive song?

Though we couldn't understand the content, the process was clear: to be a child, to play and to sing. We considered how the number 9 is found in myths connected to mysterious things from other worlds. We also knew from Peter's dreams that his feminine sensitivity was surfacing. The key to life for Peter was perhaps the very act of living magically (as seen in the number 9) and connecting to people (the new Zurich tram system) with feeling (tram stops were Helen and Amy). His discovery seemed to be the experience of eternity, of expressing himself openly, ecstatically, and joyfully, as naively as a child would, without adult inhibitions.

I remembered an early childhood memory he had told me when I had asked him if he could recall a dream from his childhood. His earliest memory was this:

> I was lying in bed in my parents' room on Sunday morning, and my two sisters came in and jumped into bed with me. What a great atmosphere!

The first childhood memory or dream is a pattern of our personal myths. Living the childhood myth in reality must be the new plan. Sandy's friend and Amy are the momentary representations, in his tram vision, of his childhood memory.

I knew from my previous work with the dying that frequently those who were thought to be clinically dead saw great visions.[2] These visions revealed secrets to them in their sleep and comas that were usually forgotten later. Why do we forget the magical keys?

The death experience ends our ordinary thinking. In dying, we achieve a great perspective, we see ourselves from above, so to speak, lying dead below. It is as if we can finally say to ourselves, "There I lie, a fine woman or man who has done this and that. There I lie, dead or dying. And why not? Here I am now, in the midst of this new and amazing experience, discovering what I always needed to know about existence."

Many of these clients had immense feeling experiences in which the secrets were given. What they got was not a new agenda for life that could be recalled and that needed to be followed, but an indescribable and, in some cases, content-less but joyous feeling of connectedness that could only be lived. Indeed, one of the secrets to life is to fully experience it.

·Our theorizing and meditating came to an abrupt halt. We looked at our watches. We thought we had been chatting for minutes but had been talking and taking notes for almost an hour. I guess we, too, had been in an altered state!

5

THE SPIRIT IN
THE BOTTLE

Remembering Peter's playfulness, we ran to the gift shop just as it was opening at 6:30 A.M., and bought him two toys, a metal truck and a furry little mouse.

We arrived in his room with the toys and found him half asleep, coughing. We wondered whether to work with him and wake him more or let him slumber. Since his cough would not let him sleep, we worked with his breathing by coughing with him. He was making slight grimaces as he coughed and we tried to help him complete them by making the faces we imagined were behind his signals or symptoms. At first we coughed exactly as he did, and then added a few extra noises to his message. We intensified our faces until he responded by making faces back. He picked up our attempts to communicate by adding to our auditory expressions. As the noises and faces increased, the cough soon disappeared and transformed into a song. He began to speak, saying it was great to be able to talk. We offered him our gifts but had to wait before talking to him.

THE BOTTLE

PETER (*smiling*): Hey, listen, listen. The problem is that the bottle is just too small for the inner life! It's just too small. Two times thirty centimeters too small!

I noticed that his actual body was intensely swollen. His kidneys had failed, and the water had been collecting with no possible outlet. I imagined how it must have felt.

> ARNY: You're right! Why didn't I think of that before? The inner spirit has a rough time in such a small bottle! Well, I don't know what two times thirty centimeters means, but I can tell you, Peter, the size of the bottle is no problem. None at all!
>
> PETER: No?
>
> ARNY: No. I know how to repair that. We can just open up the top of the bottle and let the spirit out a bit.

To my surprise, Peter picked up my suggestion and responded enthusiastically.

> PETER: Yes, let's do it!
>
> ARNY: I'd love to meet that spirit. Let's take out the cork.
>
> PETER: Where is the cork?
>
> ARNY: Hmmmm, where is it? Where? Where could it be?

Peter thought for a moment, then pointed to his throat.

> PETER: In the throat, of course. Yes, of course. We can open up the bottle, of course, Yeah. (*yelling*) And then what?
>
> ARNY: Just what you're doing. Yell and scream, of course.
>
> PETER: Yes, *exactly*. That's exactly right! *Wow!*

Then he began to shout just for the sake of shouting. We screamed and shouted together for a long time, stretching the limits of the hospital's clinical regulations and enjoying ourselves immensely. After five minutes, Peter was able to urinate again. He then asked for some fresh oranges and a dark beer.

HOLISTIC THINKING

Peter's kidneys began to function again, and he felt better. The buildup of water in his body due to kidney failure had given his inner spirit the feeling of being confined in a bottle.

Process theory tells us that the spirit in the bottle is the organizing story of his physical life.[1] Physiologically, too, the kidneys behave like a "cork" for body water when they do not function. The throat reminds us of a bottleneck and, when constricted, acts like a cork for the breath.

The experience of opening up the cork by yelling and screaming connected impressively with the opening of the kidneys. Amplification of somatic messages and comparison of these messages to dreams indicate that dreams and visions pattern proprioceptive experiences, organizing body behavior. If visual and feeling experiences change, the body changes as well. Thus, as the corked-up body experience or bottled-up vision was transformed by opening up, the body changed too. Visions, dreams, and myths use our physical bodies as a dramatic stage upon which the individual organs are actors. (See Appendix.)

Apparently, it was this spirit in the bottle making rattling noises through bronchial pneumonia and blowing up the body through kidney failure. The spirit wanted freedom. The feeling of freedom Peter experienced through yelling loosened the cork, and his kidneys opened up. Not only did his physical body loosen up, but this previously quiet, reserved, and inhibited man yelled, screamed, and roared with laughter.

REGAINING HEALTH

By ten that morning, Peter no longer required his oxygen mask, and the symptoms of pneumonia had cleared up. His lungs no longer made noise, and his blood pressure and temperature were back to normal.

The doctor who had wanted to administer morphine the night before came in for his regular visit.

PETER: Doctor, nice to see you. Seen from the medical perspective, I would say that I am in perfect health again. Don't you agree? I feel fantastic. I no longer have any pain, and I can breathe freely.

The doctor looked at Peter and looked around suspiciously at the rest of us. He seemed upset by what he saw.

> DOCTOR: Yes, but what has happened here cannot be explained by medical science. Who took off his oxygen mask?
> SANDY: My husband did that himself.
> DOCTOR (*looking at me*): But do not forget that I am the one who is responsible for his medical treatment!

And with that statement, the doctor turned and left.

CASPAR, THE HERO

Amy and I now continued to play with Peter. We tried drawing with him, but he seemed uninterested. We tried to engage him using the toys we bought for him. We showed him the truck, but he looked the other way when he saw it. Then we introduced him to the furry little mouse. He rolled over in bed, grabbed the little mouse, and hugged it. I took the mouse back for a moment and said, "Peter, this mouse is a magical mouse. It has the special property of being able to do anything its owner wants."

Peter then took the mouse back, played with it, and gave it back to me.

> ARNY: Listen here, little mouse, I now want you to do anything Peter asks. And listen now, let's see. Your name must be, must be . . . your name will be . . .
> PETER: Caspar!
> ARNY: Caspar? Caspar! You are Peter's ally.

Everyone clapped with enthusiasm. The nurse came in to check Peter's temperature, but Caspar the mouse, in the hands of Peter, interceded.

> PETER (*as Caspar*): I am doing Peter's work for him. I want to say hello to you, dear nurse, and to give you a little kiss behind the ear. Don't be shy. Come a little closer and take me in your hands. Love is nothing to fear.

The nurse turned red, not knowing how to deal with this unexpected and unusual situation. Peter explained delicately that she didn't need to be shy, for the mouse would never hurt anyone.

This was the beginning of an intense love scene with everyone Peter encountered. The mouse, feeling braver after his first adventure in this world, took stock of the situation and courageously marched forward to meet the increasing number of visitors drifting in and out of the room. The furry gray creature went out into the world to meet the relatives, nurses, and doctors.

At one point, as Amy gave Caspar a kiss, Peter said, "Hey, how about me?" Amy shyly kissed Peter, and Caspar was finally put aside. Peter now began to do the hugging himself. Gently Peter encountered the people coming into his room. He took them into his arms and looked lovingly and deeply into their eyes. His room had become a healing place for the needy and tired. Freed from his earlier "adult" identity and social status, Peter became as compassionate, wise, and innocent as the Divine Child.

Peter turned to Sandy, and they embraced. Sandy said softly, "This is the most beautiful moment in my life." Peter responded, "This is what life is meant to be." With one arm he hugged Helen, Sandy's friend, and with the other he embraced Sandy. His lovingness showed us all how to love each individual in a special way, without taking anything from anyone else or creating jealousy. He loved a single person and the world with the same arms.

It was now early afternoon. Amy and I had been there sixteen hours. I was thinking about getting back to my practice. I had already canceled the appointments I had scheduled with clients for that morning. Peter noticed my fatigue and guessed what I was thinking.

> PETER: Arny, you want to go back to your practice, but you cannot go yet.
> ARNY: But Peter, I really have to go, I need to see others.
> PETER (*meditating and deciding something*): Go. Return to your practice.

He gazed into my eyes for what seemed like a small eternity. He reached out toward me, and we embraced.

PETER: So much has passed between us, so much that is beyond words. But we must also try to formulate this in words . . . I love you deeply, and am so thankful to you. I will continue working on myself with you and with the doctor. We will get together again, soon. And . . . please take care of Sandy.

As we hugged, I cried. I mumbled good-bye as best as I could, aware that this might be the last time I would see him in this form. And then I left with Amy. I wondered how he would continue to work on himself, and how he wanted me to care for Sandy.

Later, Sandy told me that he spent the rest of the day singing, playing, and loving. He told her and others over and over that it was the most wonderful day of his life. Sandy said it was the closest they had ever been.

That day he was no longer upset about being ill. He felt well again. At midnight he said he was tired. He asked the nurse for half a sleeping pill and fell asleep. He awoke briefly some time later, and then fell asleep for the last time.

CLOSING RITUALS

The next day, Amy and I heard about Peter's death. We made our own little ceremony for him. We visited him in our fantasies and imagined that he was there with us in our living room. We both had visions in which he returned to life as a very sensitive doctor. We had no way of knowing whether these fantasies belonged to us or to Peter, yet we definitely felt better after this personal ritual.

The next night Amy and I visited Sandy and her close friends at home. Sandy was both depressed about losing Peter and elated about what they had experienced together. I was delighted to find Caspar—the mouse—enjoying life in the hands of the eldest boy.

At Peter's funeral, the minister struggled with Peter's lack of interest in organized religion. He said that God had appeared to Peter in the form of his lust for love and life. I think this was right. If Peter's dreams and final experiences had been included in the funeral service, the speaker would have said that the secret of life is living it fully and wholeheartedly. I felt that Sandy, Helen, Amy, and I had witnessed a great secret. I wondered if and how we could share those incredible events with others who had not been with us. I thought of my own death and the deaths of those I loved.

A huge group stood somberly around the grave. Peter's young daughter tossed an empty matchbox with a picture of a ship she had drawn on it into the earth. Was she aware of the archetypal journey the dead make to the other world? The eldest boy threw in a toy watch so that his father could keep track of this world. The other boy put in the shield of a warrior. Perhaps Peter would need that to face the unknown.

Peter left behind him an ecstatic experience and a lot of family work to be done. Today Sandy continues to follow her interest in psychology and is helping others to make difficult transitions. She went through many mood swings over the following months, mourning the loss of Peter, picking up her earlier interests, continuing her own learning and loving process, and building upon the foundation she had created with him. There is much more to say about her experiences, but that is Sandy's own story.

6

WHAT IS DEATH?

Before discussing the philosophical and technical aspects of work with the dying, I must pause and ask, Was Peter's experience unusual? What is death?

A thirty-year-old man dying of AIDS gave me an answer. After coming out of a coma, he said to me, "Tell people that processes have a beginning, a middle, an end, and then another beginning. Let everyone know this. And in the end, we all get a birthday cake."

This man had been in a painful dreamlike state. He had always been shy and introverted, but after coming out of the state he began to lecture to me about death. He said, "Everyone is pregnant with death. Everyone needs it. Near death, we all have the same chance. We all have the chance to become our total selves."

PERSONAL MYTHS

What does it mean to become our total selves? If I think empirically, becoming our total selves must mean living out our personal myths. Peter's early memory of his two sisters playing in his bed on Sunday morning was a mythical pattern. At the end of his life, he was sitting in bed with Helen and Sandy. We can consider the possibility that his childhood dream was the pattern of his death.

A man dying of ALS, a disease marked by progressive loss of muscle control, had a childhood dream of a sunny room. When we worked together, he stopped fighting his symptoms long enough to feel them. When he could finally make a picture out of these feelings, he had a vision of a warm, relaxed, and smiling Buddha. Then he immediately remembered the sunny room he had dreamt of as a child.

This man had been a very extroverted, physically active man who loved outdoor sports. Now, in the late stages of his disease, he was in the midst of a very meditative, quiet process. He actually felt encouraged by what was happening. His beautiful childhood dream was repeating itself. In a state of profound relaxation he worked on himself, and his emotional and physical situation improved.

One conclusion to be made is that what we call "terminal diseases" and death are personal myths trying to realize themselves.

DEATH AS PART OF LIFE

Death is a personal experience, something that is different for everyone. Every time you think you are going to die, whether it's a fantasy, a wish, or fear of an actual physical ailment, you are trying to practice dying.

Dying can be a healthy experience. One need only imagine it. The way you are needs to die. Our identities want and need to die periodically. If your identity becomes too rigid, if you have stopped growing, or if something new wants to happen, then your old self dies. At any stage of life, therefore, death is rapid change, growth, and transformation of identity.

To know about death, we have to die. My feeling is that we should practice it as a meditation, especially if we fear it. Do not wait to die, but do it now. Lie down and die. Notice what stops when you die. Notice what wants to begin.

ON FACING DEATH

Many therapists encourage their dying clients to face the reality of death, even when there seems to be little initiative on the part of the client to do so. Modern therapists make programs out of facing death, in part because we have spent so much time denying its existence.

An open or "beginner's" mind follows events as they occur, and does not recommend anything. Peter, like many people, never overtly "accepted" death. Several days before he died, his process was to fight death. Remember how he yelled, "Shit Leukemia!" Just hours before his death, he felt well and believed that he was recovering. Like many others, he did not accept death, because, in a way, he really wasn't dying. What we call death was for him a part of life. For him, death meant to live and become interested in life and loving.

When they are right near death, most people forget it entirely. There is a story that the Russian writer Chekhov drank champagne with his last breath. At his death, Jung asked for the best bottle of wine from his cellar. Near death, existence goes on and death often seems irrelevant. People go on living. Is this because life is fullest when the spirit is free?

Thus it could be that people avoid the reality of their deaths not only because they don't want to die, but also because some part of themselves is just beginning to live and is not going to die. One part of their identity is not connected with space and time. Hours before his death, Peter said he was going to continue working with me, but he also asked me to care for Sandy. Peter experienced part of himself as dying and part of himself as going on with life.

The term *death* implies a new process. It means we should begin cleaning up our present situation as best we can and moving on with the new process trying to happen.

DEATH DREAMS?

We should be careful about interpreting dreams as if they indicate death. Since I am uncertain about the meaning of death, I do not find it in dreams. A man dying of cancer dreamed a month before he died that

> the five Tibetan points in my lung area would live forever though the rest of my body was going to die.

In Tibet, death is but one state in the midst of an ongoing process of life, death, and life again, from one body to another. This man's dream shows that the part of him located in his breathing area (similar to Peter's spirit in the bottle) lives forever and another part of him (the bottle itself) is forgotten.

A seventy-year-old man dreamed:

> I am at my own funeral. I try to talk to my friends, but they are fascinated by my dead body in the casket.

We might think that this dream implies that life goes on after death. This could well be the case. In my experience, however, such a dream does not even indicate that the person will soon die. This seventy-year-old man lived another twelve years after the dream! Thus, the dream indicated that he was upset about the death of his normal personality, his career, and the associated loss of his friends. Every time we make huge changes, we die, and our friends change as well.

Death is a concept that we need when we are ready to complete something or detach our focus from it. When we have completed it or detached our focus from it, whether or not one physically dies becomes irrelevant.

WHY IS DEATH SO LONELY?

People near death are aware of the importance of human warmth. In the dream above, the friends cannot relate to the man in his altered state. The reference to "my dead body in the casket" is a description of an altered state, an identity different from the normal, working world. The man himself had never had much relationship to himself when he was not working or relating normally. He had never asked anyone else to relate to him when he was ill, sleepy, or drunk. Therefore, in such unusual and altered states, he felt and was alone.

Most of us repress states that do not go along with our accepted identities. Thus we never ask others to relate to our most shadowy spots, to our trancelike and comalike conditions. This is one of the reasons why even the most outgoing people often feel lonely. A part of them is unknown to themselves and left out of their contact with others.

We need to learn how to share our altered states with others whom we love. If we don't, when we finally enter these states we are alone. The end of our life is then an exaggeration of the loneliness we have always felt. We have no contact with others in our altered states.

FEAR AND PREPARATION

Our fear that dying will be catastrophic and nightmarish is largely due to our feelings and dream figures that we have not dealt with. The monsters we fear most can be met with before the end of life through working with dreams and body symptoms. We need to know and live all parts of ourselves now, both our angels and devils, rather than wait for the end to discover our magnificent tricksterlike natures.

Working hard on oneself, however, should not be made into a dogmatic program. Self-knowledge is not the only way to prevent difficult experiences, painful death, or suffering. Preparation for death can happen spontaneously in the last moments of life, as it did with Peter. Even if, like Peter, we do not work on ourselves and are not interested in psychology, when it becomes necessary, given the proper support and encouragement, we may suddenly pick up and follow our own processes. It seems to me that most of us have an innate ability to do so.

DEATH AS A SPIRITUAL PATH

In India, a person entering the life stage characterized by renunciation goes through a ritual of death and burial that detaches him from his family. He becomes symbolically dead to his family. Many real deaths may be related to detaching from personal relationships. Death can be a ritualistic parting from our closest friends, a way of freeing ourselves from the bottle of conventions and beliefs that we have created around us.

Death, therefore, is a concept that is useful to our normal life, to our identity with a given physical form and a specific cultural definition of being human. Death is a Cartesian, Newtonian, and in some senses mechanical idea that expresses not only the extinction of the real body, but our detachment from our old selves.

GRIEVING

Death often seems more difficult for the living than for the dying. Our feelings for the dying are intense and complex and change radically from one moment to the next. Some people refuse to grieve. Others must not grieve, but need to get back to their own tasks in life. Still others grieve for what seems like an eternity, suffering the pain of having lost contact with a loved one.

A lot of mourning and grieving can also be due to uncompleted relationship experiences with the deceased. Most of the time, we are stuck in a specific kind of relationship with them and cannot get to deeper, eternal aspects of our connections. Thus our old relationships bind us. We cannot let the deceased go, but remain sad or angry because we have not found that precious something we were seeking to experience with them.

We may also grieve because we realize that we, too, are going to die. We are reminded of our own mortality and our own deaths. We mourn because we realize that we are not now living the way we need to. We are forever putting off our own lives.

Grieving when a friend or loved one is in a coma may relate to our inability to communicate with the person in that state. This problem can be solved by our learning how to do so. We imagine the dying person to be going through pain and turmoil in their coma, but in truth we have no idea what is happening in there. Thus we need to learn to relate to people in altered states. There is no substitute for this dimension of relationship.

Grieving is often relieved by connecting to the dead person as if they were an inner part of ourselves. Believing that they are gone and unreachable keeps that part of ourselves at a distance. It is a certain way of keeping ourselves split.

Those of us left behind feel bad because we can no longer see the others, here and now. This challenges us to find out more about our own deaths, about what needs to die and what needs to live, and relieves our dying loved ones as well. Being able to connect to our projections on the dead and dying, to our own immortal selves and to eternity, can partially relieve our grief. My grieving for Peter abated when I discovered that he was a part of me, a spirit in myself insisting upon wakefulness and love.

PART TWO

THEORY AND TRAINING

7

ALTERED STATES
AND COMA

One of the basic ideas of this book is that there are powerful, dramatic, and meaningful events trying to unfold themselves in comatose states. One reason for the dramatic power of comatose events is certainly the innate drive for self-knowledge possessed by people like Peter and John. It seems to me that all of us share this drive.

The style of the individual therapist, however, may also promote or inhibit the unfolding of such trance processes. Above all, beliefs, past experience, and training contribute to determining how deeply and thoroughly we can help people near death to dive down and return with new life.

Thus the second part of this book is devoted to learning how to work with people in altered states and comas and how to understand the unusual experiences they encounter.

BACKGROUND PARADIGMS

The governing idea behind my work is a mixture of scientific realism, phenomenological respect for individual experiences, and the suspicion that everything that happens contains the seeds of our totality.[1] This latter belief makes me a modern alchemist. Whereas the early alchemists worked on transforming matter into gold, the matter with which I work is the client's perception. I tend focus less on the content of what a person says, and more on the emotional and intellectual spirit or energy of the person.

Like all alchemists, I am a believer in nature and a spiritual person. The hundreds of people I have encountered in extreme states have shown me that hidden in the most impossible or absurd conditions is something wondrous. I see human nature as a deity, for in the most confusing chaos one finds the seeds of creation.

My theory is that the interventions required for a given person in a given situation can always be found in the processes occurring. Amplifying the total process and working with perceptions bring people the feelings, insights, and relief they seek. But in order to find these interventions, we must be able to differentiate what we perceive.

PROCESS STRUCTURE AND ALTERED STATES

Process theory attempts to deal with events in neutral terms, without dividing them into matter and psyche, mind and body, conscious and unconscious. Thus the same theory and associated tools are used in a variety of psychogenically oriented states, regardless of their connection to metabolic or structural brain pathologies. Learning process work in normal situations is helpful for work with the dying, and conversely, work with the dying is excellent background for understanding normal states of consciousness. The states that dying people go through are similar to the states found in ordinary process work. Only the intensity and wonder are greater. It seems to me that nothing happens in a coma that is not trying to happen to people all the time.

Comatose states, however, do differ in specific ways from other states. Coma is the deepest form of unconsciousness. If consciousness stands at one end of the awareness spectrum, then coma stands at the other end, with the many forms of altered states in between. Coma is an extreme form of life in which the individual can almost never be aroused to respond to noxious influences. We have seen, though, that special forms of communication can enlighten this dark hole of life.

Comatose states differ from psychogenic disturbances such as catatonia in that the former are almost always connected with organic lesions or metabolic changes in the brain.[2] Process work with comas first involves relieving any possible causes creating the coma, such as glucose and oxygen deficiencies (especially with diabetics and in near-death situations). Only after the individual has been treated for organic lesions is it possible to focus on behavioral signals.[3]

COMA AND TRANCES

All states of consciousness that are different than the ordinary ones with which we identify ourselves I will call *altered states*.[4] In normal states people are capable of giving verbal or nonverbal feedback to questions and can talk about the same everyday realities that interest others.In altered states, such as those we encounter in dying processes, feedback to questions about everyday realities is diminished or absent. People cannot enter and leave these states easily. They seem absent, their memory may be disturbed, and they usually have poor space and time orientation. The duration of such states depends to a great extent upon our ability to communicate with the person.

Let us say that *normal reality* is the world agreed upon by consensus opinion. This is the world to which our normal identities are connected, our everyday life. In this world we are able to give more or less immediate verbal or nonverbal feedback if we choose. In this state we express some degree of interest in the rest of the world. Thus we can say that when Peter said to me the last day of his life that I could go back home and that I should care for his wife, he was in a normal state of consciousness.

Quarter trances describe those states in which feedback to communication is slightly delayed or unrelated. Hence, we are in a quarter trance when we are sleepy or occupied with something internally. Most of us are in quarter trances when we relate to others without wanting to.

Half trances are states in which feedback to communication is strongly delayed or very unrelated to the stimulus. We still have the feeling of connecting to the other person while we are in half trances. When writing or doing something strongly internal, we are usually in a half trance relative to the outer world. Half trances can usually be given up if need be. Half trances often occur when we listen without wanting to and our eyes become glazed and unfocused.

Three-quarter trances, also known as *semicomas,* may be related to organic problems. In this state people cannot seem to control their swings between half and full trances. This state is common for people coming out of comas or passing between waking and sleeping. The difference between the lesser trances and the three-quarter trance is that in the latter we have immense difficulty speaking about anything, especially about this world. We can be reached only with difficulty by others.

Trances, or *full comas,* are profound states of apparent unconsciousness where one cannot respond to any verbal or nonverbal approaches. Total comas may be induced by slight or seriously traumatic organic disturbances. If you scream at or pinch a person in a coma, you will not get a normal response.

First Exercise

To understand trances experientially, I would like to invite you to try the following exercise. This exercise can be done alone or with another person.

If you work alone, do this exercise as an internal series of pictures. Imagine yourself lying down and pretend that you are in a deep trance or coma from which you cannot be easily awakened. Getting into a deep trance state is easy, and it is equally easy to come out of it if you tell yourself that you must come out of it in three minutes. Trances are always just below our threshold of consciousness, waiting for us. We can feel them many times during the day.

If you work with a partner, let your partner sit next to you and simply hold your hand. Both of you simply note the kinds of experiences you are having. It is important for the sitter to say when the three minutes are up. If you are working alone on yourself, this is the end of the exercise. If you are working with someone else, then switch roles, without talking. Do the same with your partner for another three minutes, and then share the experiences that you had.

Many people who have done this exercise were surprised to note what a pleasure it was to be in a deep trance with someone else there. Others noted how lonely it was to enter into a deep state and to have another person nearby who seemed to have no connection to the state.

Some of those sitting by noticed that they felt distant from the person in the trance. Others experienced frustration at not being able to care for the person. The one in the trance also felt frustrated to discover how insufficient simple caring was. Such experiences are the goals of this exercise.

Most caring professionals have a hard time entering the world of the patient. Just being nice is sometimes not enough. Once we learn how to work with people in comas, our increased sensitivity will show us how insensitive simple nursing and caring can sometimes be! The ordinary helper deals with the comatose patient as an ill person who cannot care for himself or herself, not as a physical and spiritual being in the midst of working on the inner self to whatever extent is possible.

Since we are insensitive to our daily altered states, we ignore them in others. Neglecting our deepest innermost experiences makes us lonely. Such insensitivity may even drive us into early death or coma in order to experience our totality in peace without the disturbances of our "normal" insensitivity.

Thus coma is a trance from which the person cannot be

easily aroused. In a coma, breathing is disturbed. Breathing is generally noisy, because the soft palate in the mouth is paralyzed and the tongue gets caught in the mouth. The heartbeat is frequently strong and often variable, and the unconscious state is usually associated with apoplexy, stroke, or some other disturbance to the brain such as hemorrhage, blood clot, or (especially in children) high fever. Comas may also be connected to diabetes mellitus, Bright's disease, alcoholism, cerebral tumors, meningitis, insulin overdoses, or opium or carbon monoxide poisoning.

Brain and Mind

There is no simple connection between organic brain disturbances and coma, since not everyone with an organic brain disturbance has the same degree of trance. Psychological factors determine how our processes organize themselves around organic problems. The brain and the mind are not exactly the same. A useful analogy that fits many people with brain injuries is that the brain functions like a television set and the mind like the television station. A disturbance to the set means that we cannot get sound or pictures even though the sender (mind) is working.

The case of Dan is a good example of this analogy. After a severe stroke, he was totally paralyzed; nothing moved except his tense, shaking left arm. When we amplified the movement of this arm (such movement work will be explained in greater detail), his coma lifted as he responded with eye movements and facial expressions in conjunction with our interventions. He let us know that there was a lot happening within him even though he could not express himself adequately.

Coma Vigil

In a "coma vigil" one or both eyes remain open with minimal or no detectable evidence of responsiveness to outer stimuli. This happens with acute organic brain syndromes and is often related to cerebral accident or infection.

Ron, for example, lay totally paralyzed in bed after a brain operation for cranial bleeding resulting from a fall during a bout of heavy drinking. To the medical observer untrained in process work, he appeared to give no noticeable response to anything in the outer world. One of his eyes remained open in a comatose vigil, but even this eye did not at first respond to what was in front of it. As we began to amplify and follow his breathing and chest sounds, his eye began to follow events around him, and his breathing pattern changed, particularly in response to our recommendation to shut both his eyes and sleep if he needed to.

Those who remain in persistent vegetative conditions are understood to be brain damaged or "brain dead." Such patients are the object of an intense controversy today. Should they be kept alive? This debate will be discussed in greater detail in chapter 12. For now, I must answer this question with a simple "yes." I will show that people who are still breathing should be allowed to live. We need to learn how to communicate with them and give them the chance to make their own decisions about life and death.

8

WORKING WITH COMAS

Working with a person in a coma can be seen as a form of refined communication. It is an intimate relationship in which the therapist helps the person in this state learn how to work on and communicate with himself. We are helping or teaching the person to reflect, meditate, and value altered-state experiences in order that they may become self-healing and elucidative.

Thus the lessons we learn from working with comas will be applicable in all of our relationships. Until now, mainstream psychologies have focused primarily on understanding altered states. Now we must develop the tools to enter these states, communicate with those who are in them, and come out of them again. If comatose and trance states are not helped to complete themselves, they freeze awareness into a kind of void that some clients have described as a "whiteout" or "blackout."

GETTING OFF THE WHEEL: THANATOS ETHICS

One client of mine told me after coming out of a coma that he had had the experience of being tied to a huge revolving wheel. This image resembles the Tibetan wheel of fate and becoming, which symbolizes everyday life, compulsion, and lack of detachment. For me, psychology is a way of getting off this wheel for a moment, discovering where you are, and making a conscious, wakeful decision about whether you want to get back on that wheel or not. Using our awareness, we can process the events that are happening to us. Otherwise, we are passive, unconscious witnesses of our fates.

Process work with the dying leads us to a position that I referred to earlier as Thanatos ethics. This ethics—which I will discuss in detail in chapter 12—is both a philosophical viewpoint and a practical method for getting off the wheel by allowing us to make our own decisions about life, decisions that would otherwise be made by others. Embracing Thanatos ethics means that we create the awareness necessary to process experiences and decide the future of the body.

TRAINING EXERCISE

Up to now, the best method I have found for learning how to process trance states is to study them, to practice working with people in trances, and to experience being assisted by someone else while you are in a trance. We have covered enough theoretical ground at this point; what is needed now is experience and practice.

The following exercise develops some of the tools we need to work with trances. Read through the entire exercise before trying it. If you feel uncomfortable about trying it, you may want to be the "sitter." Decide whether you will do it alone or with someone else. Whenever possible, I think it is best to try this with someone else.

Pretending to be in a trance is just like being in one, except for the fact that you have made a conscious decision to investigate your awareness. Thus this experiment will give you an experience of your own trances and help you to process those of others. We should also remember that trances are normal occurrences: we all have them many times a day! Working on them now is not only a chance to process near-death experiences, but a chance to process what happens to us every day as well.

GETTING INTO A TRANCE

One person chooses to be the "client"; The other one is the "sitter." The client lies on the floor or in a bed and is asked to act as if he or she were in a coma or deep trance. (If you work alone, see yourself going into a coma, and see yourself simultaneously as the sitter.) If you work in pairs, you will need about thirty minutes for this exercise.

PROCESSING THE TRANCE

Your process work begins by *connecting* with the comatose person. Sit near your "client." When the client exhales, speak gently and slowly, in the rhythm of his breathing, near his ear. Say something like the following: "Hello. I am Arny. I am really here with you today. I am going to speak with you and in a moment I will also gently touch your arm. . . . Now this is my hand on your arm. You can feel me pressing gently on your arm. This is a way of being with you."

Now gently touch the client's arm as he inhales and relax your touch when he exhales. Continue, following the rate and strength of the breathing. You press on inhalation because you are matching his breathing energy with your strength. (One can also gently touch the upper part of the chest, the lower part of the leg, or the top of the head.) Remember to speak unobtrusively and gently, and yet close to the client's ear when he exhales.

The way you relate nonverbally is as important as what you say, since the client understands you with body feeling as well as with hearing. Communicating congruently means getting a verbal message across in such a way that it matches your nonverbal message. Congruent communication is believable communication. The client's breathing rate matches the experiences he is having in his trance. Thus speaking and touching him at the same rate means that you are communicating with him in his language, or on his wavelength, so to speak. Thus he is likely to have the impression that you are where he is.

Many people in persistent vegetative comatose states or trances will respond to you by giving you minimal cues or feedback. Minimal cues can be seen through changes of breathing rates or eye and mouth motion in connection to your communication. These cues may indicate that the client is responding to what you are doing. Such responses are welcome positive indications that you are making contact.

I recently visited an eighty-year-old man in the hospital after he had been totally paralyzed by a stroke. I said to him very quietly and gently, in conjunction with his breathing rate, "Hans, you and I are going to have an important experience with each other this evening." Most comatose clients need at least twenty minutes to respond, but this man's response was so rapid, it shocked me. His eyes instantly opened. He focused and looked directly into my eyes. As I communicated with him, he continued to give me cues with his eyes, leading me from one experience to another.

The second step in processing the trance involves *finding the way*. Here you should make a statement about your intentions. You might say, for example, "I am following the rate of your breathing. I want to follow everything that happens in you. What goes on outside and inside of you is important because it will show us how to proceed. It will show us the way."

Telling the client that inner processes can guide us gives the client the idea that what is happening is important, that there is a way that can be followed. It also gives the client the feeling that he is not alone on this path; you will provide help to follow the path. And finally, this message enables and encourages him to become aware of himself.

I recommend that you gain access to the "way" by helping the client follow specific signs and signals. As he exhales, you might say, "All you have to do is to notice what is happening. See whatever you are seeing, if you are seeing. Feel everything you feel. Hear the things you hear, if you are hearing. Take all the time you need, and see, hear or feel."

The third step in this work requires that you begin to *pick up minimal cues*.

You should now give the client time to respond. While you tell him to hear, feel, or see what is happening, watch for any of the following minimal cues:

- *Auditory changes* in breathing rate, depth, and sound.
- *Movement changes* in spasms, twitches, jerks, facial movements, or grimaces. Some clients suddenly move the corners of their mouths, enlarge their lips, or move their eyebrows together as if they were thinking about something. If these motions occur consistently after a stimulus, you may consider them forms of interpersonal communication (in contrast to primitive nervous reflex actions).
- *Eye changes,* as in opening the eyes, focusing them, or directing the gaze. Eye color may also change. Some comatose patients' eyes may be open and glazed, indicating that they are not looking but feeling or hearing something instead.

It may take a while before the client responds or before you notice some of these minimal cues. While you continue to follow the client's body motions and breathing, do not just be passive, but participate by observing what is happening inside and outside of yourself. You may become aware of changes in your own breathing, changes in body temperature, or even the appearance of spontaneous fantasies or plays of imagination.

I remember once being at the scene of a car accident. I was sitting near a severely injured man waiting for the ambulance. I suddenly had a vision of him leaving his body lying dead on the road. The next minute he stopped breathing. I spontaneously became very angry with him. "Hey," I said. "Don't do that now! Take your time!" He began to breathe again and survived.

The kind of response you give to a minimal cue is important to the client. Your responses indicate that you have connected. He knows now that he has found you. Your responses also help him to become aware of what he is doing, and will help him to "say" more.

In initial process work, the most useful kind of response is the blank access response, one that encourages the client to communicate further, yet does not assume what the content of the communication is. Trying to understand the client intellectually may inhibit his or her expressions, which if given enough support will clarify themselves.

Not at all incidentally, we use blank accesses all the time. Meditation, staring at the sea or mountains, or even listening to music are all blank accesses—means to open up to whatever needs to arise. We fill in the blanks with our own sounds, images, and fantasies. All blank-accessing methods are soothing and creative because they help bring up what is inside by giving it space and time. A verbal blank access would be, "Oh, yes, that." An auditory blank access would be to say, "Listen to that." Such encouraging yet empty statements can be very useful. A visual blank access like "Look inside and see," or "Look at the blank wall and paint a picture" can work like magic.

When working with the comatose, it is important that you respond with verbal statements that are enthusiastic but whose content is vague. If the client's eyes focus, then you might say, "Oh, I see that, too!" Statements such as "Look at me!" are too directive and may not correspond with what the person is actually viewing. Blank statements of enthusiasm such as "Wow!" "Yes!" or "Gosh!" are interpreted by the client as he needs to. If the eyes move from one side to the other without focusing, you might experiment with a statement such as "I hear that, too." Or, if he closes his eyes, relaxes, and looks sleepy, you might say, "Feeling things is important," or "Quietness is lovely." Every time you say something, be certain that you also communicate the same message through your hands by gentle changes in your touch.

Blank Movement Access. If the client moves even a little bit, then you might say, "Oh, what a lovely movement!" Again, just noticing or commenting on what the client is doing is an encouraging act, which doesn't direct or confuse by assuming what the content might be.

A useful way to encourage movement is to gently touch the muscles from which a movement originates. In the case of large-scale movements of the arms and legs, it is useful to help the limbs move or to gently inhibit them from moving. (Remember Peter? When I gently resisted his leg motion, he completed it and yelled, "Shit leukemia!") Help create and support the motion from where it originates by gently using your hand on the body to extend, contract, relax, or excite motion in the direction in which it is already going. You need to use a very developed sense of touch and motion, for you are working with anatomical elements moving in reference to deep, unconscious, and dreamlike inner experiences. If your work is on the right track, the body will respond by moving with or against you. If you are off the track, you will probably get no response at all.

Another way is to gently touch a limb or hand that seems to have implicit motion within it by placing your finger on a bone—for example, a wrist, elbow, ankle, knee, or the head. Such very slow movement allows the client to become aware of his own movement potential. He can then "direct" you with his muscles without having to have the strength to move the entire limb alone. The important thing is not your motion but the client's direction. Once that person's own motion is found, a statement such as "Yes, yes! Go on with that movement" helps him express himself in movement. In this way, a slight spasm of a finger can turn into a bird's flight, as one woman later told me.

If the limbs remain completely flaccid, your movement work is not getting any response. You are in the wrong communication channel. If they are very stiff, do not try to change the rigidity, because it is there for a reason. Try encouraging it with statements such as "You are using your strength well. Go ahead and use it." One woman woke up when I said that and said, "Yes, I know the way. I'm now going to take it."

Breathing Accesses. Another very useful mode of communicating with someone in a deep coma is to breathe along. Pace the client's breathing for two or three breaths, and then add another kind of breath, your own kind, with a different sound or tempo to it. Some clients respond strongly to this kind of communication by adding on to their breathing new sounds, rhythms, or noises.

These methods of finding the way, responding, and communicating nonverbally are tips to help you carry out this exercise. Take about fifteen minutes per person. The "client" should act as if in a coma, and the "sitter" should pace his or her breathing, look for minimal cues, and then respond. Go back and forth between "speaking" and "listening" with all your senses.

Minimal Feedback

Almost everyone responds, although people who are taking painkillers will need longer to respond than those who are not drugged. If you have not noticed any response, go back and repeat your recommendation that the client see, feel, or hear whatever it is he's experiencing. If the eyes open and look at you, don't assume that he wants to relate to you. Do not ask questions that require an answer. If someone looks at you, then just look back. You might just say, "It is a pleasure to be with you." I would not speak too much or attempt to relate. Remember, he has possibly entered a coma in the first place to go within and to focus upon himself. Let him respond the way he wants to. Accept whatever he has to give now.

There is something mysterious about this work. Following processes whose content is unknown is an act of faith, a belief that the individual knows and will show us the way. Working with blank accesses is working with something we do not know. As long as someone is alive, I assume that that person has a purpose in being here that he or she knows and is reacting to. Focusing so intensely on minimal cues is a form of worship and love, so to speak. We are using everything we have and making something out of almost nothing.

9

COMA AND SHAMANISTIC EXPERIENCE

To date I have not met anyone who has not responded to the kind of interaction described in the last chapter. Being encouraging, interested, and gentle will suffice for minimal communication with most clients. Others, like Peter, will want to go even deeper. What happens after the comatose client begins to respond is a form of process work that borders on the ordinary forms of psychotherapy described elsewhere.[1] This chapter therefore concentrates on the details that are necessary to help people complete their momentary journeys.

PROCESS IDEAS ABOUT ILLNESS

We need to know that the kinds of feelings and thoughts we have about the comatose person strongly affect him. A medical attitude toward the person's experiences and the belief that they are due to pathologies can affect his reactions and even, under certain circumstances, make him comatose again. For example, one man who was recovering from a brain injury became ecstatic when he looked at an inner picture of "ripping and crashing." Then his doctor came and said to him, "Now Joe, remember that you have had a brain injury. You are in the hospital recuperating. Today is September 17, 1987. Look at the calendar." Joe's response was to become very foggy and to complain of a severe headache.

To use terms such as "ill," "psychotic," "deranged," "comatose," or "drugged" can be considered an aggressive act that cuts people in altered states off from their experiences. We need to know that these terms are consensus-reality descriptions of internal and unknown processes. They are our way of dealing with what we do not understand.

A phenomenological approach accepts the comatose state as it is described and allows the signals descriptive of this state to unfold into a process. Thus, when Peter started to cough near the end of our work with him, this "coughing" was not only seen as a symptom of pneumonia, but understood as a potentially meaningful state trying to express itself. The cough turned into yelling, and later the noises became the spirit in the bottle asking for freedom.

DURATION OF COMATOSE STATES

A coma is understood by the terms in which it is expressed. It is not only a mental illness, or simply an organically based condition. It is a trance state, one of many states of consciousness in an ongoing process.

In my experience, the amount of time spent in a trance or coma depends upon the client's belief in what is happening. The greater the belief, the less time it takes to complete the state. Peter's coma was shortened in part because of the ability of those around him to appreciate his state. The nature of the coma in the case of John, the man described in chapter 1 who had been unresponsive for six months, was partly due to the inability of those around him to process his groans and moans. The length of his coma was proportionate to his inability to unfold the story of the angels driving the ship.

It seems to me from the many cases I have worked with that the duration of comas is usually not connected to unfinished business in the client's life, except as this touches upon unfinished internal work. Peter, for example, needed to free his spirit, and this in turn changed his outer life. But what does "outer life" mean? John's inner work with the angels changed his outer life too. He went on vacation.

CHANNEL WORK

Following processes means relating to experiences in the modality in which they are expressed. For example, there may be *visual modes*, such as John's vision of a ship of angels or Peter's vision of the Zurich tram system. Before she died, my mother was amazed by a very bright star. Others might see dead relatives, guides, or wise teachers. When people perceive their experiences visually, speak to them in visual terms. Encourage them to look at the forms, colors, lights, and so on.

The *breathing* of comatose people is an auditory experience containing much information. Peter's singing and celebrating came from his rasping cough. Work with auditory signals by listening to them, mirroring or repeating them, or even adding your own noises to the sounds.

Some of Peter's apparently irrelevant *hand motions* were signals that led to his directing our singing, like a symphony conductor. His movements needed encouragement. In another case, a sporadic head movement to the right indicated that the woman was looking at her imagined husband-to-be. The arm spasms of a young child dying of brain tumors were the beginning of a hugging process. In fact, in many of the comatose states I have seen, the movement signals have developed into some process of hugging, touching, and loving.

Some people have *telepathic experiences* and sense they are in various other places. They experience their bodies flying above the ground, though the body seems to us to be in agony. We must be careful not to guess what a comatose person is experiencing. It is rarely what we expect. Many *body feelings,* too, are incomprehensible to the outside world. Our interpretation of visual and auditory signals such as facial grimaces or coughing almost never coincides with the comatose person's body feelings, for our interpretations are based upon our experiences with normal neural connections. The comatose person may experience herself as smiling, though we believe she is making an angry grimace.

Semicomatose people may sense that the world is torturing their body. I have frequently seen this feeling connected to the hospital staff's negative attitude toward the patient. Some personnel do not understand inner experiences, or feel that the patient is exaggerating her situation. Occasionally such pain may be due to inferiority feelings or anger toward authorities. I remember a young AIDS patient who suffered from terrible stomach pain. When he got angry at me, growled, and told me how to be a better therapist, he felt better.

In a comatose state, people usually do not experience much pain because they do not identify with their normal bodies. (I will explain this more completely in the following chapter.) Coming out of the coma, they feel pain again as they resume their old identities. When pain is present, it is because we need to feel it for some reason. I remember one woman who mumbled from a partial coma that she was a powerful leader. When she came out of the coma and back into her normal identity, she complained of having been in pain for months. I recommended that she go back and feel her pain, and then make a picture out of the feeling. She did this, and in her vision she saw the origin of the pain: the "devil" with a pitchfork! I then told her to think devilish thoughts. She smiled, but said she couldn't do it because that would mean being too powerful. In her coma, she was able to identify with her power, but in her normal identity this power was forbidden to her.

Pain indicates that we need to integrate the pain maker. The pain creator is a part of our psychology we need. If we do not pick it up consciously, it hurts us. There are many ways to reduce pain by processing the figures that create it. We should be careful, however, about recommending to everyone to psychologize their pain away. Some people may not be successful at psychological work because they need to be more dependent upon others, or they may need to ask for medical help. In addition, without the availability of some form of process work that integrates pain, medication must remain a preferred treatment.

We frequently and incorrectly project onto dying people that they are in pain. To check whether or not the projection is true, ask the client if he or she is in pain. Suggest a binary (yes/no) method of responding by moving a finger or an eyebrow or by changing the rate of breathing.

RELATIONSHIPS

Feeling issues in relationships are important to people near death and in half and three-quarter trances. In a coma, however, or a peak state experience, relationships frequently entail experiences of universal love or feelings for the whole creation. I remember one woman to whom I said good-bye for the last time. I told her how beautiful she looked. She responded by looking at me, at her nurse, and at the others present, and then said, "Aren't we all so magnificent!"

In more normal states, we need some form of relationship work to process issues with relatives and visitors.[2] The ill person wants to complete unfinished issues or experiences happening in a couple or family. I remember one man who could not die. He was worried about the financial security of his girlfriend. He asked a priest to marry them so she would get social security benefits after his death. A few hours after the ceremony, he died.

Parapsychological and telepathic experiences are also not uncommon. Many dying people have told me that they have lain in bed and simultaneously walked around in other cities. Such cases lead me to the idea that awareness can also be located outside of the physical body. Our awareness can be located at the particular place on this earth and in time that corresponds to our present state of development and psychology. Thus, for example, a man in one city with an unfinished relationship in another city was able to tell me about objective events (which I verified afterward) going on in that city. When he finally confessed his love to the woman in that city, he was at peace.

It is clear from such examples that the psychological state of the dying person determines their physical location. I remember my mother saying to me just before she died in Miami that she would soon meet me in Zurich, where she wanted to study. Hours before his death, Peter said he would go on working with me. These statements are processes that extend outside of the time and space of the real body.

Many people speak of going home. One woman said she wanted to go home to her mother. "Let's go," I said. She repeated over and over, "Going, going, going home." She was blocked from going to her inner home. I took a lucky guess and said, "Can you smell your mother's cooking?" "Soup," my client answered. "Chicken noodle soup." Going home meant going to the familiar, to this woman's real self. Home was where she had come to birth, where she could grow up. So it was not surprising when she soon said, "A new, bright star is born. A star!" "Be a star," I responded, "and show us where to go from here." The star was eternal wisdom, which poured out of her in expressions of love and knowledge.

It is important to remember that the person in a coma is not the same person or in the same state of mind as before. Therefore, relationship problems and disagreements may no longer be important. One woman sitting with her dying father angrily told him that he had not been loving to her during his life. His response was that neither he nor she was real. If you have unfinished problems with a comatose person, I would suggest that you work on them internally, understanding your feelings for the person in the trance as a part of yourself.

The outline of comatose events can sometimes be seen ahead of time in dreams, as in Peter's case. The final love scene of his life was predicted in his dreams. His coma was an attempt to drop his ordinary self and to identify himself with the dreaming world. This process differs from other situations in which we inadvertently split off parts of ourselves, experience them in our dreams, or find them in our body symptoms, while remaining in normal states. The coma allows total immersion. Perhaps that is what death is: total immersion in some original dream.

COMING OUT OF COMAS

When we come out of a coma, we retrieve our old personalities as well as our old bodies. Thus old symptoms may reoccur. For example, a woman who was comatose following a severe asthma attack had vivid experiences of being a child. As she was coming out, the child disappeared and a chronic cough turned up. When we worked with the coughing, out came the child again! The coma can be the solution to symptoms because during a coma, the individual is able to unconsciously identify with the process behind a dream or symptom. Yet a coma is not a complete solution because the process happens so unconsciously that integration is extremely difficult.

Some people who come back from near-death experiences speak about them willingly. Others come back only partially from such experiences, and stay in a half-trance until they die. They respond to your questions only when you adjust your communications to their language. It is as if they are saying, "Thank you for making me conscious of where I am, but I would like to stay here." Some patients actually prefer their altered states to ordinary reality. This is even true of patients who had earlier indicated that they would prefer death to a semicomatose state. For us in our ordinary state of consciousness, it is practically impossible to imagine that a coma could be an ecstatic state that one might not want to leave.

I have noticed that people who come back from comas too early, without processing their experiences in depth, will seek a way to return. One client of mine had been in a coma connected to a terminal disease. He suddenly and spontaneously recuperated and jumped back into his normal life and concerns. He did not think at all about what he had experienced in the coma. He soon developed mysterious dizzy spells and as a result was in a serious automobile accident in which he was knocked unconscious. After he recuperated, we worked together to reaccess the accident. He began to play the role of the force that had put him in a coma—in the latest case, the tree he had driven into. The tree said, "Go back into the coma. Free yourself from your mortal concerns." This discovery had a great impact on him, and he decided to pay less attention to his financial security and career goals, and to risk living more of his own creative desires. This need for a new lifestyle, I imagine, had been at the core of his coma.

TRANCES AND SHAMANISTIC EXPERIENCES

In some parts of the world—in Bali, for example—trances and comas are cultural rites. People go into trances for personal reasons and for collective ones as well. A whole group can go into a trance in order to act out and solve problems. Religious experiences frequently occur during strong trances because the freedom from an old identity opens one up to divine experiences and cosmic feelings.

Peter's trance and awakening were part of a resurrection. His enlightenment and rebirth from a coma remind us at least in some small way of the resurrection process of Jesus Christ. Just before the resurrection Jesus cried out to God in agony and despair, "Why hast Thou forsaken me?" Peter's last powerful exclamation before his coma, "Shit Leukemia," was not all that different from Christ's cry.

Before the death of our old personality, we identify ourselves as the victims of nature. After the "death" of the primary process (that is, the way we identify ourselves) we have a chance to resurrect and connect to more universal and cosmic experiences such as love.

Deep trances may also occur with people in the midst of life. I remember one woman who entered a trance doing body work. She focused for some time on the subtle motions in her body. She began to experience herself as God and could not come out of her trance until she overcame her inner resistances to having religious experiences. She told me later that some inner father-figure was trying to tell her that having feelings was just crazy.

I recall another woman who had always been very adapted and sweet. In a trance following a dance experience, she became the opposite, the Greek monster Medusa: intense, violent, and direct. Other strong trance experiences come to mind. I remember a shaking woman who entered a movement trance that she came out of after dancing. She imagined herself to be the divine Shakti, dancing for the whole world.

DROPPING THE HUMAN FORM

Trances scare us and can even make us feel crazy if we do not have the inner tools to help us live, understand, and integrate them. When a trance is fully processed, it always gives rise to more life, not less. Up until now, the development of such inner tools has been mainly limited to meditators and shamans. I recall how don Juan, the Mexican shaman in Carlos Castaneda's work *The Second Ring of Power,* informs his budding apprentice that the purpose of his training was to learn how to maintain his awareness in altered states, to "dream" and "see" and eventually develop to the point where he could drop his human form. According to don Juan, not every warrior lived through this immense transformation, but those who did could not longer be identified with their old selves.

Most powerful trances and many comatose experiences create this transformation experience, which don Juan calls the "end of the human form." Peter literally dropped his old personality and became a new man. Until I heard about the parallel between coma experiences and the training efforts of don Juan, I had felt that process work with comatose clients was probably an isolated beginning of a new set of experiences.[3] Now I am even more encouraged than before in my work, since I understand that many—perhaps all—of us attempt near death to make not only immense changes, but a revolution in our personality. With more research, we may well come to the conclusion that the dying process is one of many attempts to recreate the human being.

REACCESSING TRANCES

One of the themes of this book has been that death experiences also happen in life. Thus the trance states which occur near death can occur at any time in life. It seems important to me to process these trances by learning how to reaccess them or bring them back to consciousness. Such work is made more difficult by our fear of what we may do in such trances. For example, epileptic trances, that is, so-called grand mal attacks, are often unconscious processes that enable the sufferer to be violent. Thus the fear of such trances and seizures can be connected to unknown anger. As long as the unknown factors remain unconscious, trances tend to reoccur or persist.

To reacess a trance, it is often enough merely to ask the client to act out what they experienced in the trance. If she is afraid, then it is sometimes helpful for the therapist to model the trance behavior by acting it out first. A completed trance process seems to inhibit its reoccurrence. I remember a woman who had persistent fears of death and frequent attacks of what she called "spaced-out dreaminess." She felt drawn to another world, and when given the chance in a seminar actually "left" for that world. She became blue in the face, had visions, spoke excitedly about the stars, and after hours of work decided to live on earth as long as she could keep in touch with her journey to the stars. This decision altered her view of life and marked the end of her "dreaminess" symptom and fears of death.

Up to now only shamans have been able to leave this reality, to enter altered states through dance, drugs, and dreaming, and to return with messages for us all. Now it seems that comatose people are attempting the same sort of shamanistic feat. The more we learn about these feats, the more we shall learn about living completely and bringing together the various worlds we encounter.

10

DREAMBODY AND MYTHBODY

Comatose states and near-death experiences contain a virtual kaleidoscope of body experiences. The various experiences one may have in a coma go by such names as "real body," "subtle body," "astral body," "ethereal body," "the double," "out-of-body experience," or "end of the human form." The term used to describe any one experience depends on the specific body feeling and the cultural belief system of the person.

In this chapter I differentiate body experiences not by any particular belief system but according to how they are experienced. I will speak about three common body experiences: the "real body," our normal body experience; the "dreambody," a body feeling reflecting recent dream contents; and the "mythbody," an archetypal pattern of the dreambody often appearing in deep trance states. I focus upon these body states because not only do they occur near death, but each can be experienced in life.

THE REAL BODY

The real body is that body experience with which we identify. You describe your real body every time you say, "My body feels (this or that)." The real body is the body we talk about when people ask us how we feel. The real body is the body that feels fine, has a cold, a lower back pain, or stiff joints. The real body suffers from allergies, cold and heat, a fever, or a rash.

We normally identify with the real body; the dreambody is the experience that happens to us or to our bodies. For example, we often say that we feel miserable because of a splitting headache or because of an allergy. Maybe something makes me itch. I have a stuffy nose, or something is making me nauseated. These sentences show the way the real body experiences the dreambody: the splitting nature of the headache, the element that is itchy, or the thing making us nauseated. These experiences happening to us I call "dreambody" experiences, because they can always be found in our dreams.[1]

The real body experiences itself most frequently as the *victim* of the dreambody experiences. Our real body feels like the victim of altered states that are trying to get our attention, or as the victim of secondary processes that appear in the form of incomprehensible signals such as fatigue, sadness, anger, visions, and dreams. Peter initially experienced his real body as the victim of leukemia and pneumonia. The real body experience was represented in his dreams as the bridge, badly shaken by storms and needing repairs. When he went over the bridge to the other side of the river, he left his real body, the "bridge." When he said he was trembling with panic, this was the bridge, being "shaken" to pieces by storms. His first experiences of leukemia were feverish symptoms that made him tremble and shake. The real body has symptoms; the dreambody is the symptom maker. The real body is what carries the dreambody to the doctor.

One client who suffered from backaches dreamed about these two body experiences. He dreamed that he was an ape carrying a demon on his back to the doctor. The demon, however, was invisible to the doctor. This is just what happens in real life. We try to locate the dreambody in terms of thermometers, blood tests, and X rays. The dreambody, however, is invisible; we can only feel it ourselves and work with these feelings.

The Death of the Real Body

The real body is important to us because we identify with it. Everything we call "me," our way of life, our ideologies, and our concerns, are connected to this body. When a client tells me that he fears death, then I understand that his present identity will soon come to an end and he will begin to identify himself more with his dreams.

We die over and over, each time we connect to our new dreams. Dreams of leaving the body and visions of hovering over the body and looking down on it are experiences of the new dreambody getting a perspective on the real body. From the new vantage point, we see that the way we have been leading our lives is dying. Such dreams do not necessarily indicate that we are actually going to die, but show that a part of us is trying to grow by detaching itself from our present identity.

The Dreambody

Thus the dreambody includes all those physical sensations that happen to the real body. These are the things that bother and excite us. We usually first notice the dreambody as a disturbance to the real body. In our dreams we see it as figures or situations challenging our personal identities. In life, we may project it onto other people. Body symptoms represent the dreambody impinging on our awareness. Leukemia, for example, is a real-body description of a dreambody trying to reach consciousness. The winds and storm, the flame burning up Peter's old identity, and the spirit trapped within the bottle were dreambody signals.

Raymond Moody, a physician who has worked extensively with dying people, quotes many patients who placed their awareness in their dreambodies and who disliked their real bodies. One woman, who had clinically died and came back to life, said:

I could see my own body all tangled up in the car amongst all the people who had gathered around, but, you know, I had no feelings for it whatsoever. It was like it was a completely different human, or maybe even just an object.[2]

Another of Moody's patients said that he

didn't like being around this thing that looked like a dead body—even if it was me![3]

Michael Sabon, another researcher of near-death experiences, records many statements in which the dying distance themselves from relationships.

It was like all relations were cut . . . Everything was just so—technical.[4]

RELATIVITY AND PAIN

It is necessary to think relatively about the body. Our body experiences depend upon our viewpoint. If our viewpoint is located in the real body, then, as victims of the dreambody, we suffer pain. But only *part* of the personality is in pain. If insight, inner work, or spontaneous change switch our identities to our dream figures, then we are in our dreambodies and, as such, have no pain. This is why the woman above could look down on her real body, which was dying, and feel nothing.

Thus if a client can identify with the dreambody, the wind, the fire, the storm, then—much to our surprise—the experience of pain disappears. This is what happened with the woman I described in the last chapter who was in constant pain, which, however, disappeared when she identified with the devil, the dreambody who was making pain. When we become the origin of pain, we integrate it. When Peter identified with the spirit in the bottle instead of with the bottle, he not only freed himself from pain and coughing but also from his old inhibitions. When he became the stormy winds of panic or fear, then he was not the victim of sleeplessness or fever, but the source of energy behind these symptoms.

DREAMBODY AND MYTHBODY

The symbols of the real-body and dreambody experiences can always be found in recent dreams or fantasies. Likewise, the body feelings associated with the real body and dreambody can always be felt in our momentary feelings.

On the other hand, some body experiences are just over the threshold of our ability to feel them. We can feel them, however, if someone massages or touches pressure points on the body surface. All body sensations that need special help, methods, drugs, and techniques to be felt, I call "mythbody" because the pictures and stories associated with these normally inaccessible feelings are fantasies and dreams with archetypal and impersonal origins.[5]

For example, if, when you work on a headache whose pain is readily accessible, you find a pressure behind the headache, chances are there will be a similar pressuring figure in the recent dream. The feeling, and the associated dream image, are acute and readily accessible. If, however, you feel well, but when massaging your head you find a point that seems sore, the stories and images that come in association with the feeling and pain of this point will be less familiar than those in recent dreams. For example, after pressing the point, you might have a vision, as one of my clients did, of someone piercing you with a sword and declaring battle. My client did not have a recent dream about such a figure or battle. He had to go back to childhood to find a dream about such a situation. The point that hurt, as well as the vision and associated memory, was beyond the threshold of his normal perceptions.

The mythical imagery connected to body experiences over the threshold of awareness is more impersonal than imagery associated with acute symptoms. One woman who worked on such a point felt the pain to be like a hammer. She saw a vision of a god with a hammer, insistent and demanding. These visions were completely foreign to her. She had never heard of the Germanic thunder god, Thor. While real-body and dreambody images and feelings are acute, readily seen and felt, and somewhat familiar, myth-body images and body feelings are less accessible, not readily seen or felt, and usually unfamiliar. Furthermore, while the dreambody is often connected to momentary unconscious feelings, mythbody experiences are usually connected to immense archetypal tasks. The mythbody is a creator body, timeless and free.

Peter's vision of the key to life and of the spirit trapped in the bottle are both mythbody experiences in that they do not have personal associations like familiar dream figures. Rather, these mythical images are associated with transpersonal life. His mythbody wanted freedom from his ordinary body. It was involved in great tasks, in loving, freedom, and healing.

Many diseases, including various forms of cancer, are mythbody diseases, because their beginning stages are rarely felt. The feelings are inaccessible; we may not even dream about them. Entering this deep, inaccessible realm of feeling and vision through deep body work connects us to the distant mythical part of ourselves and gives us a chance to live our mythical tasks. Thus any form of deep body work that connects us to the mythbody's almost inaccessible feelings and images is the beginning of preventive medicine for insidious diseases as long as the experiences unraveled by body work are processed. Certain forms of massage and hands-on body work may heighten awareness of buried experiences in our musculature or inner organs through the use of special hand pressures and motions.[6] Certain drugs (such as LSD) can also connect us to the mythical realm but may have the disadvantage of disturbing our ability to process these states in detail while they are happening.

THE SPIRIT IN THE BOTTLE

Let's look at the mythbody experience of the spirit in the bottle that Peter had the morning before his death. Did he know the Brothers Grimm's fairy tale called "The Spirit in the Bottle?" (For a more detailed version of this tale see the Appendix and my earlier work, *Dreambody*.) In that tale, a young man, forced to leave medical school due to lack of funds, hears a spirit calling for freedom from a bottle lodged in the roots of a great tree. He frees the spirit, which turns out to be threatening and vengeful. But in the end, the spirit gives the young man magical medicine that heals all wounds.

I somehow detected this mythbody in Peter. He told me that he had once been interested in studying medicine. But like the fairy-tale hero, Peter too had run out of funds. He subsequently lost interest in medical studies and gave up the life he had been leading.

The spirit in the bottle is vengeful and murderous, for it has been locked up too long. It wanted eternity and ecstasy, not the mundane tasks of today and tomorrow. Once freed, the spirit can heal. Remember how Peter told the doctor that from the viewpoint of medical science he was healed? Peter's immediate symptoms really did disappear. His bottle, his body or lifestyle, was too narrow for his fiery spirit, which needed freedom to complete its tasks.

We all have a spirit in the bottle. How much time and space does any of us give our spirit? Is it free to do what it needs here and now?

11

THE IMMORTAL YOU

Dreambody and mythbody analogies are found in the death theories of such highly developed ancient civilizations as China, Egypt, and India, as well as in Western research on death and dying. These theories give us an extended sense of the journey we may go through near death and of the developments that are trying to happen now, in the midst of life.

TREATMENT OF THE DEAD BODY

Whereas Indo-European peoples kept the corpse in the house for extended periods of time, partially embalming it, other early peoples buried the corpse in or near their homes.[1] Some cultures thought the corpse could still have sexual intercourse with the living partner. Others felt the corpse was a representative of the dead spirit; it was alive and had to have a tube near the head in its grave so that it could still breathe and eat.

There is an almost universal ancient belief that the dead body contained the living spirit, and the Egyptians seem to have gone the furthest in actually performing rituals for the spirit of the dead body. In their instructions for the rite of mummification, it is written:

Then anoint his head twice with good oil of myrrh and address him: "O, Osiris, the oil of myrrh which comes from Punt is put upon you in order to enhance your aroma through the god's aroma. The secretion which is upon you comes from

Re, and it comes (in this way) to beautify (you). . . . Your
soul walks on the land of the gods, upon your body. Horus is
on you, he who comes from the myrrh oil, out of Osiris.[2]

After the entrails are removed to be mummified, and the
head is bandaged and anointed, the mummy is then ad-
dressed again:

"Your head comes to you so that it will not be separated
from you: it comes to you and does not separate itself (from
you) in eternity. . . . The clothes of the gods are put upon
your arms and the splendid robes of the goddesses on your
limbs, so that your arms will be strong and your legs powerful . . ."[3]

The body of the dead person is equated with a mythical
figure, the divinity Osiris, whose soul must be reminded to
keep its head, as it becomes part of the sky, the underworld,
and the temples on earth. This recommendation fascinates
me. When the body is in a coma, or even apparently dead,
it is important not to "lose one's head." In other words,
the ancient texts stress the importance of maintaining
awareness in altered states, for this awareness can determine the length and outcome of a coma, or rather, the way
in which the "dead" person continues to grow.

DIFFERENTIATED DEATH EXPERIENCES

Religions and belief systems differentiate the path of the
dead. The land of the dead was often thought to be full of
dust and worms, clammy and dark. The Hel of the Teutonic
world, the river Mictlan of the Aztecs, and Hades of the
Greeks are all characterized in this way, as is Sheol, the
gravelike abode of the dead in the Old Testament.

While commoners, evil people, or those murdered in a
specific manner went to the dark places, the enlightened
and chosen ones went to a lovelier beyond, above the
ground. In dark Hades as described by the ancient Greeks,
there were no doctors, priests, or saints. Those initiated
into the Greek mysteries went to the glorious Elysium or to

the "Islands of the Blessed." The fallen warriors of Germanic myth were taken to Valhalla. Aztec warriors and women who died in childbirth did not go to Mictlan but followed the sun across the sky.

If we understand the doctor, priest, or warrior as symbolic of an awakened consciousness that has met and processed its perceptions and problems, then we can understand more easily why the "common" aspects of ourselves are left in hell. Lack of awareness and insight into our perceptions turns them into a "bad trip." They become the impossible and incongruous demons of hell, the spirits that disturb our equilibrium.

REAL BODY, MYTHBODY AND DREAMBODY

Our real-body concept is roughly equivalent to the Chinese *Po*, the Egyptian *Ka*, or the Indian *Ahamkara*, all concepts of an individual soul. These spirits are said to remain near the physical body at death. The afterlife spirits known as *Hun, Ba*, and *Atman* from the same three cultures are said to free themselves from the body in the grave and leave for transpersonal, independent realms, free of the previous, personal identity. They are similar to our mythbody concepts.

Death Body Theories

PROCESS CONCEPTS	WEST	CHINA	EGYPT	INDIA
REAL BODY	Real Body	*Po* Soul	*Ka* Soul	*Ahamkara*
DREAMBODY MYTHBODY IMMORTAL BODY	Out of Body	*Hun* Soul	*Ba* Soul	*Atman*

Chinese, Egyptian, and Indian concepts differ from process concepts. Yet comparative cultural studies give us a perspective upon dream- and myth bodies. Across many cultures, beliefs about death and afterlife reveal a twofold structure that is similar to our ideas of conscious and unconscious. The body that is thought to hover around, beneath, or near the physical body is what I call the real body because it is related to our identity. The other spirit, that with a transpersonal life, which is capable of leaving the physical identity and flying to the stars, like *Ba, Hun* or the *Atman,* is closer to the mythbody since it is detached from personal identities.

THE UNIFICATION OF THE BODIES

The goal of existence, in many cultures, was not understood as death. Afterlife processes were supposed to continue until the different spirits united. Thus the *Ahamkara* or ordinary ego in Hinduism marries the *Atman* and creates the *Jivan,* that is, the united person who wanders throughout incarnations. As the *Ahamkara* part of the *Jivan* changes through incarnations, the *Jivan* changes too until it escapes the cycle of birth and death altogether and is free. Likewise, the Ba attempts to unite with the Ka, and the Hun with the Po, to unify and transform in other worlds. While the Hun, Ba, and Jivan souls strive for detachment and awareness, their physical analogues, the Po, Ka, and Ahamkara souls strive for reconnection with the earth, rebirth, and fertility. This reunion with the earth through reincarnation is considered desirable in many cultures, but according to Tibetan and Indian belief reincarnation is to be avoided.

These speculations correspond to my empirical observations that at the point of death some, like Peter, experience their mythbodies in ordinary life and die, while others return to their everyday jobs and continue living and working.

THE IMMORTAL BODY

The unification and transformation of the soul bodies can already be seen in the dying when personal psychology begins to mix with transpersonal, timeless, and archetypal experience of what I shall call the immortal body. The experiential domain of all four bodies (real body, dreambody, mythbody, immortal body) is summarized in the following table.

Body Experience Spectrum

	REAL BODY	DREAM-BODY	MYTH-BODY	IMMORTAL BODY
Imagery	the body	recent dream figure	big dream or saga	etheric body
First body description	upset	symptom	nothing unless aided	distant feeling
Processed body experience	victim	creator of symptom, no pain	sense of purpose, no pain	freedom, wholeness, completeness

The viewpoint that we take determines what we see. When we observe ourselves in our ordinary state of consciousness, we are in the real body and feel impinged upon by other body experiences. If we work with the body and create these pressures, we find ourselves having images of recent dreams. In this case, we identify with or are in our dreambodies and may feel disturbed by our real bodies. When we work with the feelings that are at the threshold of awareness, then we are in our mythbodies and look upon the real body with detachment, as if standing on a mountain looking down at ourselves in the valley below. When we begin to live closer to our myths, we experience timeless immortality and freedom.

RESURRECTION AND THE IMMORTAL BODY

According to medieval Christianity, the dead person was believed to become resurrected in Christ; the resulting resurrected body was "pneumatic," that is, a combination of spirit and flesh. In the Pauline tradition this metaphysical body was imagined to contain the essence of divine qualities of the individual in a timeless manner. The immortal body was a state in which the essential information about the personality of the deceased was conserved. In more scientific terms, the immortal body was thus imagined to be a sort of information field or "body" symbolized by the appearance of the living person.

We find this same idea of an immortal field in the ancient Egyptian belief that Osiris's grave was the mysterious place from which new life could arise again, the place from which a new world could be recreated. This mystery was, at the same time, an "image" imagined to be in the body of the deceased.

These ancient beliefs express awareness of a universal truth about our bodies. If we think of the empirical work described in earlier chapters, then we will recall that the dream images arising from body sensations (such as the spirit in the bottle) strive for realization and literally pattern the reawakening of the individual.

EMPIRICAL EXPERIENCE OF THE IMMORTAL SELF

If there is a principle of conservation of energy and information at all stages of life, it seems likely that the process we see happening near the moment of death continues after death. This means that archetypal patterns such as love and learning go on after the death of the body. Here I would like to postulate an information field that tends to organize people and events into specific patterns. Whether this field reappears as a given person or as a group idea depends upon the individual and the times.

The purpose of this speculation is to stimulate further research. Personally, it is important for me to stay close to what can be experienced in the moment. Those readers interested in a hint of what the immortal body may feel like might try the following exercise:

1. Pretend that you have been alive for many centuries. Imagine that you transform in some way after death. Can you picture yourself as a spirit that will be here for eternity? Have you ever dreamed of such a figure? Can you remember a figure that would represent this timeless self? Make a picture out of your immortal self.

2. Make some slight movements that this figure might make. Notice how these movements differ from yours. Can you move a little bit like this figure and still see yourself at the same time?

3. Now try to feel the body feelings this figure might have. Can you locate a part of your body that feels like this figure? Now look at this part, feel it, and move like it all at once.

4. Ask this part of yourself a question that has been bothering you and to which you would like an answer. Ask it now and wait for an answer. Take your time.

5. If you receive an answer, notice the effect it has on you. This immortal self has the maturity and wisdom that you need.

Now that you have some experience of this immortal personality, perhaps the following will make sense to you. The immortal self is the Self, the larger personality behind our dream- and mythbodies. Our ordinary and mythical dreams, symptoms, and trance states are all aspects of this larger personality, what Jung would have called the Self. This is our wisdom center, the greater being behind the personal one. The more we become our total selves, the more we come to resemble this figure, the more it becomes our double. It is this immortal Self that appears near death from the cocoon of our real bodies lying in a coma. Our earlier selves have now become too small for the immortal experience.

When working with people who are dying, it is helpful to imagine this immortal body, for then we can understand the otherworldly comments that they may make. We are talking to their immortal selves, parts that we now know to be in ourselves as well. Peter said, ''What we have experienced is beyond words, . . . but we must attempt to formulate this too.'' This was his immortal, wise Self talking.

One of the reasons why it is so important for us to know the immortal and mythical part of ourselves is that we need to integrate it, to enlarge our lives with it as much as possible. Doing so will make this world numinous. Without connection to the immortal Self we will feel, as we often do, that life is just not worth living.

Some of us may fear our wise and detached sides because we imagine that getting too close to this immortality will result in a loss of connection to our younger selves. Just the opposite is true. Most young children live in full experience of the immortal Self; that is why dying is often easier for them than it is for adults. Death and time are adult, social concepts, not realities for young children. In the mind of children, people do not die. Thus Peter's children gave their father gifts for the new world. As adults, we all—including those who hate their mortal bodies and want to leave this world—need to make more contact with our immortality—not less—for only then will life be worth living. The immortal part of us evokes the sense of knowledge we once had in childhood, in the womb, or in some mythical Eden. This is precisely the exciting addition we need to bring into our mundane lives.

We all know that we shall die. In fact, at certain times we all want to die. Far from thinking this wish absurd, we need to realize how intelligent it can be. We have forgotten our essential nature under the pressure to be who we are not. This idea of having forgotten our essential nature runs through philosophy, Eastern and Western scriptures, and prophetic poetry. Every religious source seeks to reawaken this forgotten self-knowledge.

RELATIVITY AND DEATH

Death is relativistic. From the viewpoint of our real bodies, death is a tragedy, a loss. From the viewpoint of the mythbody, death does not exist. From the psychodynamic view, death comes when something new is trying to happen and is split off. If we experience the inner figure representing this new element, our grieving abates as the concept of death disappears. When we integrate spirits they leave.[4] Whether we die in a Newtonian grave or live in a numinous planetary field organized by the physics of nonlocality depends upon the position of our awareness. In fact, whether we live or die depends upon our point of view.

This can be seen in the story of the death of an old Zen master. As he was dying, his students gathered around him, sadly lamenting that this would probably be their last sitting with him. He became furious with them and demanded, "What do you think these teachings are all about? Where but right here do you think I will be going?"

The dying master, in other words, becomes a field, an idea that is omnipresent and available to all. An old dying woman, about to switch her awareness to her immortal body, had the following talk with me just before her death:

CLIENT: A child . . . a boy . . . a star is born. Why is . . . what is life? What is sickness?
ARNY: Illness is junk. Throw it out.
CLIENT: No.
ARNY: What is illness? I mean really what? Go inside and ask the star.
CLIENT: Illness is a part of us which is trying . . . trying . . . to . . . be known.

The star that was born was her mythbody. It was her mythbody that was asking these questions. Just before she died, she hummed,

> Row, row your boat, gently down the stream,
> Merrily, merrily, merrily, merrily,

and then despite her paralysis from a stroke, she heartily sang out loud,

> *Life . . . is . . . but . . . a . . . dream!*

She had made the transition in identities. Jung, too, met an eternal part of himself in one of his last dreams. He met a meditating yogi and suddenly understood that our reality was the yogi's dream.[5] Thus there is no single, absolute reality. Or, rather, reality is a mixture of eternal experience, of the immortal you and your everyday life.

12

BRAIN DEATH AND
THANATOS ETHICS

Working with comatose states indicates that in states of brain damage, there may be more capacity for awareness than we have believed possible. Extrapolating from this idea, we could say that as long as the body lives, consciousness is possible. This extrapolation leads in turn to a Thanatos ethics, a philosophy and paradigm of dying that recommends

1. refining methods to help people in altered states connect to their own inner awareness
2. allowing them to make their own decisions about life and death

At our present stage of medical science, we question when the life of a comatose person ends. Today, the medical community responsible for the individual answers this question together with the family of the dying person. Some members of the medical community think that once consciousness is gone, the person is lost. What remains is a mindless organism.[1] According to this attitude, when the brain no longer functions, there remains only a lifeless shell. The body has outlived its owner. In 1981 the President's Commission for the Study of Ethical Problems in Medicine, Biomedical and Behavioral Science proposed the Uniform Determination of Death Act, which reads in part as follows:

an individual who has sustained either: 1. irreversible cessation of circulatory and respiratory functions or 2. irreversible
cessation of all functions of the brain including brain stem, is
dead.[2]

BRAIN DEATH

Until recently, the heartbeat was the measure of life and its
absence, the sign of death. With the advent of modern
technology in medicine, however, it is now possible to
revive people whose hearts and breathing have stopped.
Even when the brain has been damaged beyond repair, the
other vital organs may continue to function. These circumstances make it imperative that we develop new definitions
of life and death. The current atmosphere in the medical
community is probably best represented by the following
statement from a classic textbook on coma:

> agreement that the brain and the person are one has essen-
> tially removed the ethical conflict that otherwise derives from
> the almost universal respect for the dignity of the individual
> human being.[1]

This opinion suggests that since the brain and the person
are one, if the brain goes, so does the mind, and hence there
is no person present. Yet this black-and-white picture, resulting from equating the human being with the brain, has
been disputed by neuropathological studies on the brains of
those in chronic vegetative states that show that injury to
the cerebral cortex is sometimes "hardly sufficient to explain the patients' premortem mindless behavior."[4]

Brain death means that no part of the brain functions. A
person whose brain is dead can be maintained artificially on
a respirator only for hours or, at most, for several days
before cardiac arrest sets in. Brain death is understood as
total nonresponsiveness, lack of movement, lack of brain
stem reflexes, fixed and dilated pupils, and inability to
breathe without a respirator.[5]

PERSISTENT VEGETATIVE STATE

In brain death the whole brain is functionless. In the common vegetative state, only part is destroyed. In this state,

> the brain stem, a primitive region that connects the brain to the spinal cord, is usually intact or mostly intact. With a brain stem intact the person is capable of stereotypical reflex functions, breathing, sleeping, digesting food, but is incapable of thought or even any awareness of the world around him. A person could remain in this state for years.[6]

Decorticate posturing and spasticity are characteristic of this state. Limbs contort and contract so that the elbows, wrists, and fingers bend toward the center. People in this state still have primitive reactions and may yawn, smack their lips, or grimace without apparent purpose. Behavior in these vegetative comas is generally assumed to be meaningless. Hence it is not surprising to hear that a number of bioethicists, philosophers, and doctors are beginning to expand the definition of death to include people in persistent vegetative states, individuals who have lost their intellect, memory, speech, and awareness of self and environment.[7]

If this is the case, however, then many like John (the man who got on the ship going to the Bahamas) will lose their life support systems without having completed their inner work. Of course, one could argue that it makes no difference since such people are going to die anyway. To this argument I would have to say that after having processed the experience of a coma, some people actually decide to come back and live! Moreover, no one knows for certain what happens once the physical body dies. Will the awareness we have now be of use to us after the body is gone?

Regardless of the above definitions, even in the case of a persistent vegetative state like John's it is clear that the mind and the brain are not the same. Therefore the determination of death must be given back to the individual and not left in the hands of those burdened by the high costs of hospitalization, nor those frustrated by their inability to communicate with the vegetative patient. Though we cannot ignore the pain and cost involved in maintaining life, we can ameliorate our frustration by learning more about the experiences of the comatose patient.

As Julius Korein, Professor of Neurology at New York University School of Medicine, said,

> There is no moment of death. The moment is a legal construct . . . Look at cardiovascular death. The heart stops. The doctor listens to the chest. Was that the moment of death? With modern equipment, you can detect signs of electrical activity in the heart forty minutes after it has stopped beating. The moment of death is a fiction.[8]

Work with comas touches on ethical questions and cultural philosophy. What is life and death? My definition is an empirical one: Life and death can be defined only by the individual, moment by moment.

I think, for instance, of Sam. He had brain stem damage and had lain in a persistent vegetative condition for weeks. Ever since a massive stroke had left him totally paralyzed, he had not responded to anyone. Sams's family was suffering from having lost contact with him. They also suffered from guilt feelings about keeping him alive, since before his stroke, he had told his children that if he ever went into a persistent vegetative state his life should not be prolonged unnecessarily.

Amy and I established immediate contact with him in his coma. After seconds, he seemed to awaken from his coma and stared us in the eyes. He was able to communicate to us through minimal but obvious eye movements. He had decorticate posturing, and so we worked with his spastic hand which soon clasped ours. I "spoke" with him through a binary communication system by gently touching his facial muscles to sense spasms occurring there in response to questions. With our help, over a four-hour period he showed minimal indications that he could learn. It seemed that with patience the spastic, contracted hand could teach the limp, flaccid one how to move.

After we established contact with him, using the mode of

communication recommended in chapters 7 and 8, Sam, Amy, and I managed to agree that Sam's facial muscle spasms could be used as a binary mode of communication. "Yes" in response to a question would be implied by a muscle spasm around the mouth, "no" would be implied by the absence of any spasm.

Finally we asked him to answer the question that plagued his family. "Do you want to live?" I asked him. He gave an immediate answer: he not only grimaced but opened his entire mouth! This clearly meant yes, he wanted to live.

Up to this point, Sam had not been able to open his mouth at all. He had barely been able to yawn. Using the same binary system, we were able to ask other questions to get yes and no answers. Sam wanted to live in order to complete an inner process. We gave him inner work methods to help him on his way. He indicated that he was in the midst of an inner trip; he was trying to climb a fantasy mountain and meet a new woman! He apparently needed some time to complete his journey, for he died only several months later.

Not everyone is interested in living. I remember Roger. I had never seen him before. He had been a chronic drinker, and was now suffering from brain stem damage and had been in a persistent vegetative state for weeks. When "asked" (using a method similar to that we had used with Sam) if he wanted to live, Roger said "no." As it turned out, his medical staff had decided, together with one of Roger's relatives and without reference to our work, to withdraw his life support system within a few days. In this situation the medical system's considerations coincided with the comatose patient's decision.

Thanatos ethics means giving each individual the chance to make his or her own decision. The future for dream work and body work near death is clear. We need to learn more about how to unfold the signals of profound states of unconsciousness, so that we can give our clients the ability to make their own decisions about life.

It seems to me that as we bring more light and awareness to altered states, the foundations of our cultural beliefs about reality will change. I guess that life will become more interesting and death less of a problem.

Comatose states are very special dreams attempting to facilitate our drive for self-knowledge. In this blackest hole of life, the processes that have been waiting inside of us our whole lives seek completion and realization. In the light of this idea, life appears to be the search for self-knowledge, for the generalization and globalization of our abilities. Thus the warm person of today becomes, near death, a divine and loving deity in the cosmos. And a romantic soul like Peter transforms into the messenger of a new form of relatedness for his city.

The present work adds a practical, almost mundane feature to what is already known about death and dying: final symptoms of terminal physical illnesses are paths to enlightenment. Body signals, regardless of when they appear, are dreams searching for realization. When these symptoms are processed, pain and morbidity are relieved, reminding us that where we live now is a fabulous place to be.

From Asian, Greek, Mesopotamian, Roman, Jewish, Christian, Zoroastrian, and Islamic traditions, we are reminded of the journey awaiting us to the forgotten Self. But now the route is a bit clearer; it sometimes wanders through the shadow of trance and coma.

However, we must not forget that many people going through these altered states need our help to realize their total selves. Indeed, they want intimate communication. Many prefer it to ordinary loving compassion. For without it, a special moment can be missed as the mind spins wildly in a turbulent river flowing to the sea.

The diagnosis of cerebral death can awaken us to working with the growth process of dying and to communicating with what we once imagined to be the afterlife. What seems at first to be a mindless body fighting the grip of time can be an attempted last ecstatic dance that creates freedom from a confining identity, and greater life, not necessarily physical death. The death that worries us now will be, from another perspective, the birth of our myth.

NOTES

1. A Big Ship

1. I use the word "process" here to indicate the psychological method of unraveling inner, unconscious experiences by following verbal and nonverbal cues that are normally below the threshold of awareness.

2. I am indebted to Ernest Rossi of the Jungian magazine *Psychological Perspectives* for recommending this name to me. Ernest also introduced me to the work of Milton Erickson and his attention to minute signals, which Erickson called "minimal cues."

3. Cf. my earlier books, which likewise derive from my experience in process work. *Dreambody* (1982) shows how dreams and visual archetypes connect to body experiences. *Working with the Dreaming Body* (1984) applies process work in case reports. *River's Way* (1985) discusses the history and philosophical background of process-oriented psychology, and *The Dreambody in Relationships* (1987) shows how process work can be used to work with relationships. *City Shadows* (1988) may be helpful in understanding the greater background to comas, and *Inner Work* (1989) discusses in greater detail many of the inner-work procedures recommended here.

2. Crossing the Bridge

1. For a more complete review of working psychologically with symptoms, see Mindell, *Working with the Dreaming Body*.

4. Coma and Rebirth

1. Communicating with patients in comas and working with pain is discussed in greater detail in chapters 8 and 9.

2. This has also been corroborated by others. See particularly Raymond Moody, *Life after Life*, (New York: Bantam Books, 1976).

5. The Spirit in the Bottle

1. *Dreambody* is another term for process-oriented psychology. It refers to the idea that fantasies and dreams are also visualizations of body experiences. For further treatment of these ideas, see Mindell, *Dreambody, Working with the Dreaming Body*, and *River's Way*.

7. Altered States and Coma

1. For a more complete explanation of the background and philosophy of process-oriented psychology, see Mindell, *River's Way*.

2. See Mindell, *City Shadows*, or any standard textbook on psychiatry for further information on comas.

3. See Plum and Posner, *Diagnosis of Stupor and Coma* (Philadelphia: F. A. Davis, 1982), for a guide to the diagnosis and treatment of coma.

4. For an overview of altered states, see Weinhold, *Altered States: An Explorer's Guide to Inner Space* (Denver: Love Publishing, 1987)

9. Coma and Shamanistic Experience

1. See Mindell, *Working with the Dreaming Body*.

2. See Mindell, *The Dreambody in Relationships*.

3. I am especially thankful to Carl Mindell for pointing out to me this reference to don Juan.

10. Dreambody and Mythbody

1. See Mindell, *Dreambody*.

2. Raymond Moody, *Life After Life*, p. 40.

3. Ibid.

4. Michael Sabon, *Recollections of Death: A Medical Investigation* (New York: Harper & Row, 1982), p. 21.

5. The reader familiar with Jungian psychology may suspect a parallel relationship between dreambody and mythbody and Jung's personal and collective unconscious. Jung's terms, however, refer to personal and archetypal associations, whereas dreambody and mythbody concepts are related to the momentary accessibility of body experiences. Thus an archetypal image may be part of the dreambody if it is already close to awareness.

6. Aminah Raheem's unpublished manuscript "Process Oriented Acupressure" (Zurich, May 1986) and Fritz Smith's *Inner*

Bridges: Zero Balancing (Atlanta: Humanics New Age, 1986) can be especially useful in this regard.

11. The Immortal You

1. For the cross-cultural phenomena referred to on pages 99–104, I am indebted to Marie-Louise von Franz, *Death and Dreams* (Boston and London: Shambhala, 1986).

2. Von Franz, *Death and Dreams,* p. 92.

3. Ibid., p. 93.

4. A family from Appenzell, Switzerland, with whom I once worked claimed they had a poltergeist that banged their shutters whenever they sat down for supper. Since the family appeared to be very quiet, I asked the daughter to bang on the table and make jokes and noises during dinner. As soon as everyone joined her, the poltergeist left.

5. C. G. Jung, *Memories, Dreams, Reflections* (New York: Pantheon Books, 1961), p. 323.

12. Brain Death and Thanatos Ethics

1. Kathleen Stein, "Last Rights," *Omni* (September 1987), p. 59.

2. Ibid.

3. Plum and Posner, *Diagnosis of Coma and Stupor,* p. 325.

4. Ibid., p. 7.

5. The brain stem controls the autonomic vegetative functions.

6. Stein, p. 59.

7. Ibid.

8. Ibid.

GLOSSARY

Afterlife. The concept of an awareness that continues to exist after physical life is completed.

Altered state. A temporary alteration of focus from the primary to the *secondary process* that may be created willfully or spontaneously through a *channel* change.

Brain death. The state in which all functions of the brain are permanently inaccessible. The body can be maintained artificially for hours or days at the most. The signs of brain death include total unresponsiveness, lack of movement, loss of brain stem reflexes, fixed and dilated pupils, and so forth.

Cerebral death. See *Vegetative state*.

Channels. The modes in which we perceive. They include the following:
Auditory: hearing and noticing information as sound
Kinesthetic: the sense of movement
Proprioceptive: noticing feelings such as pressure, heat, temperature
Relationship: noticing information as if it were observed by or coming from another person
Visual: perceiving with reference to sight
World: perceiving information as happening in or noticed by the world at large

Coma. A state of extreme insensibility to outer stimuli from which it is difficult to arouse the individual, connected to psychogenic problems, organic brain lesions, or systemic metabolic changes such as glucose or oxygen deficiency. The duration of a coma depends upon the extent and severity of the pathological process, the ability of the helpers to process its contents, and the psychology of the individual. (See also *Trances* and the definition of *coma* according to Plum and Posner, *Diagnosis of Stupor and Coma*.)

Coma vigil. A *persistent vegetative state* in which one or both eyes are open.

Consciousness. A term sometimes referring to wakefulness, at other times implying the highest state of awareness, one in which we are aware of what and how we perceive. According to Plum and Posner (*Diagnosis of Stupor and Coma*), consciousness is "a state of awareness of the self and the environment and coma is the opposite, i.e., the total absence of awareness of self and environment, even when the subject is externally stimulated."

Death. A relativistic term based on the observations of the *real body*, referring to the annihilation of our present identity.

Decorticate posturing. The characteristic contortion and contraction of the limbs in a comatose state so that the elbows, wrists, and fingers bend toward the center. People in this state still display primitive reactions and may yawn, smack their lips, or grimace without apparent purpose.

Dreambody. A description of the experience we have of our bodies, occurring when we relate images to body feelings and symptoms. The dreambody is usually experienced as a disturbance to the real body and first comes to awareness in the form of symptoms.

Edge. The limit of what we believe we can do. A description of something we think is impossible for us to experience or live with.

Mythbody. The transpersonal *dreambody*; a body feeling

that is usually beyond our awareness threshold. The images and stories associated with it have little to do with our everyday life but are usually connected to *personal myths*.

Nonlocality. The idea from physics that the world behaves as if it were spaceless, since certain signals can travel faster than the speed of light.

Persistent vegetative state. A state in which the brain stem, or primitive region of the brain connecting the brain to the spinal cord, is intact or mostly intact while other parts are disturbed. The person in such a state can have stereotypical reflex functions, can breath, sleep, and digest food, but is thought to be incapable of thought or awareness of the environment.

Personal myth. The generalization of a childhood dream or memory that becomes an organizing factor in the creation of lifestyles, chronic symptoms, and issues. It may also organize the last experiences in life.

Primary process. Everything that is connected to our personal identity.

Process. The flow of signals in *channels* over short periods of time, and the changing experiences of identities throughout a lifetime.

Processing. Working with signals or bits and pieces of information, or allowing them to unfold.

Real body. Our primary body identification. The experience of being a victim, being in pain, or being the recipient of things happening to us on the outside.

Secondary process. Experiences that we do not perceive as belonging to our personal identity. We perceive them either as happening to us, or as emotions and experiences we are reluctant to identify with, such as viruses, anger, fear, power, and numinosity.

Semicomatose state. A condition of apparent insensitivity to the environment in which the individual will occasionally mumble in response to communication from others. (See also *Trance*).

Signals. Bits and pieces of information.

Trance. Any alteration in our normal focus, differentiated into four states. In a quarter trance our feedback is slightly delayed and unrelated. In a half trance feedback is strongly delayed or very unadapted to the stimulus, but we still have the feeling of connecting to one another. In a three-quarter trance, or semicoma, one swings between consciousness and apparent profound insensitivity. Those coming out of comas go through this state. In a total trance, or full coma, one is in a profound state of apparent unconsciousness with no response to verbal and somatic stimuli that are not adjusted to the patient's inner experience.

Unconsciousness. The state of being identified with perception, i.e., being unable to be aware of, notice, or follow perceptions.

Vegetative state. According to Plum and Posner (*Diagnosis of Stupor and Coma*), a vegetative state is a

> condition that sometimes emerges after severe brain injury and comprises a return of wakefulness accompanied by an apparent total lack of cognitive function. An operational definition is that the eyes open spontaneously in response to verbal stimuli. Sleep-wake cycles exist. The patients spontaneously maintain normal levels of blood pressure and respiratory control. They show no discrete localizing motor responses and neither offer comprehensible words nor obey any verbal commands. . . . In most instances the vegetative state follows upon a period of sleep-like coma.

Other terms used to describe this state are *coma vigil*, apallic syndrome, cerebral death, neocortical death, and total dementia.

Victim body. The experience of the *primary process* of suffering from symptoms and diseases that stem from *secondary processes*, i.e., processes happening outside our identity.

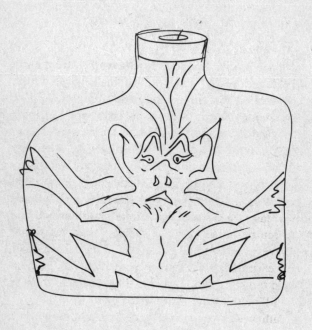

APPENDIX

THE SPIRIT IN THE BOTTLE

There was once a poor woodcutter who worked from early morning till late at night. When he had finally saved a little money, he said to his son, "You're my only child. I've made a little money by the sweat of my brow, and I'm going to spend it on your education. If you learn some decent trade, you'll be able to keep me in my old age, when my limbs are stiff and I must sit at home." The boy went away to the university and studied hard. The teachers praised him and he stayed for a while. When he had almost completed his courses, his father's meager savings were finished and he had to return home. "It's a shame," said his father sadly. "I have no more to give you, and in these hard times I can barely earn what's needed for our daily bread." "Dear father," said the son, "don't worry, I'll get used to this life and maybe I'll be the better for it in the end."

As the father was preparing to go out and earn more money cutting and piling firewood, the son said, "I'll come along and help you." "I don't know," said the father. "It might be hard on you, you're not used to heavy work. I doubt if you could stand it. Besides, I have only one axe and no money to buy another." "Go and ask our neighbor," said the son, "he'll let you have an axe until I've earned enough to buy one."

Excerpted from *Working with the Dreaming Body* by Arnold Mindell (London & New York: Routledge & Kegan Paul, 1985). Reprinted by permission.

The father borrowed an axe from the neighbor, and the next morning they went to the forest together. The young fellow helped his father and was as cheerful as could be. When the sun was high in the sky, the father said, "Let's rest a while now and have something to eat." The son took hs bread and said, "You rest father, I'm not tired. I'm going to take a little walk." "Don't be a fool," said the father. "What's the good of running around? Afterward, you will be too tired to move. Stay here and sit down."

But the son went deeper into the forest and ate his bread. He felt light and gay and looked up into the green branches, to see if he could find a nest. Back and forth he walked and at last came to a big angry-looking oak tree, that must have been hundreds of years old and was so thick that five men couldn't have girdled it with their arms. He stopped, looked at the tree and thought, "Lots of birds must have built their nests in that tree." Suddenly, he heard someone calling. A muffled voice was crying, "Let me out, let me out!" When he looked around, he couldn't see anything, but he thought that the voice came out of the ground.

"Where are you?" he cried.

The voice answered, "I'm in among the roots of the oak tree, let me out, let me out!"

The young man cleared away the dead leaves and looked among the roots until he finally uncovered a small hollow and in it found a glass bottle. When he held the bottle up to the light, he saw something that was shaped like a frog, jumping up and down inside the bottle.

"Let me out, let me out," it kept crying.

Suspecting no harm, the student pulled the cork off the bottle. In a flash, a spirit slipped out and began to grow, and it grew so fast that in seconds a monstrous fellow, half as big as the tree, was standing there.

In a thundering voice, he said, "Do you know what your reward will be for letting me out?"

"No," said the young man fearlessly, "how could I?"

"Then I'll tell you!" cried the spirit, "I'm going to break your neck."

"You should have told me that before," said the student. "I'd have left you in the bottle. But I'll keep my head on my shoulders all the same. You'll have to consult a few more people before I let you tamper with my neck." "More people, indeed", said the spirit. "You've earned your reward and you shall have it. Do you think they've kept me shut up in here all this time out of kindness? They did it to punish me. I am the mighty Mercurius, and when somebody sets me free, it's my duty to break his neck." "Not so fast," said the student, "first I've got to know that you really were in that bottle, then I'll believe that you are truly the mighty Mercurius." "Nothing could be simpler," the spirit replied haughtily. Whereupon, he pulled himself in and made himself as thin and small as he had been before and crawled right through the bottle neck. No sooner was he inside, than the student shoved the cork back in place and tossed the bottle in its old place among the roots of the oak tree. The spirit had been outsmarted.

The young man started back to his father, but the spirit cried pitifully, "Oh please let me out, please let me out." "No!" said the young man, "you can't fool me twice. When I catch somebody who has threatened my life, I don't let him go so easily."

"If you set me free," said the spirit, "I'll give you enough to last you as long as you live."

"No," said the student again, "you'll only cheat me again."

"You're turning your back on good fortune," said the spirit. "I won't hurt you, you'll be richly rewarded."

The young man thought to himself, "I'll take my chance, maybe he'll keep his word." So he pulled out the cork and the spirit came out as he had the first time and stretched and spread until he was as big as a giant. He handed the student a piece of cloth very much like a poultice and said, "This is your reward. If you put one end of it on a wound, the wound will be healed, and if you rub iron or steel with the other end, it will turn to silver."

"I'll have to try that," said the student. He went to a

tree, gashed the bark with his axe and rubbed the gash with the cloth. The bark grew together and the wound was healed. "It's all right," said the man. "Now we can part." The spirit thanked him for setting him free, and the student thanked Mercurius for the gift and went back to his father.

"Where have you been all this time?" asked the father. "You've forgotten all about your work. I told you you wouldn't get anything done."

"Don't worry father, I'll catch up."

"Catch up?" said the father indignantly, "You don't know what you're talking about!"

"Just watch me, father, I'll have that tree felled before you know it." He took his axe and rubbed it with the poultice and struck a powerful blow. But the iron had turned to silver and the blade had bent.

"Father, look at this wretched axe you've given me, it's all bent."

The father was horrified, "Now I'll have to pay for the axe, and where will I get the money?"

"Don't be angry with me," said the son, "I'll pay for the axe."

"With what?" said the father. "Can you tell me that? You may be full of book learning, but you certainly don't know anything about cutting down trees."

Later on, they returned home together and the father said to his son, "Go and sell that ruined axe. See what you can get for it. I'll have to earn the rest so that we can pay our neighbor."

The son took the axe to town and brought it to a goldsmith who tested it and exclaimed, "This axe is worth four hundred talers!" The goldsmith gave him four hundred talers right there. The student went home and said, "Father, I have got the money. Go and ask our neighbor how much he wants for the axe."

"I know already," said the father. "One taler and six groschen."

"Look, father," the young man said, "I've got more money than we need." He gave his father a hundred talers and said, "From now on you shall live at your ease and never want for anything." "Good Lord!" exclaimed his father. "How did you come by all that money?"

The student told him exactly what had happened and what a prize he had won by trusting his luck. With the rest of the money he returned to the university and continued his studies. He was able to heal all kinds of wounds with his poultice, and he became the most famous doctor in the world.

Now, can you imagine what sort of people or what cultures would dream about this tale? To begin with, the tree is, among other things, a symbol of vegetative experience, like the nervous system of the human being. Mercury would then be the wild spirit which we have bottled up in our bodies by being decent, law-abiding citizens. The father symbolizes the boy's stiffness, his teachings, his patriarchal consciousness, and the boy is the symbol of an ego which can free the spirit in the body. He is like the dreambody worker. He is you and me, who are studying dreams and body problems.

If the tale deals with a cultural problem, then we must recall that it is a Grimm's fairy tale, a tale from Europe. Europeans and Americans all have a similar dream. Our culture tells us: Be civilized, bottle up your true personality, or else let it out so quickly that you explode and go to war. Mercury is the symbol of pressure and tension, the feeling of being bottled up. He is the experience we often have of a tension headache or heart pressure, or of a stomach ache. He is a symbol of the pressured feeling everyone gets in a group which is too stiff and uptight.

BIBLIOGRAPHY

Birkhäuser, Peter. *Light from the Darkness*. Basel: Birkhäuser Verlag, 1980.

Castaneda, Carlos. *The Second Ring of Power*. New York: Simon and Schuster, 1972.

———. *Journey to Ixtlan*. New York: Simon and Schuster, 1973.

Cavendish, Richard, ed. *Mythology: An Illustrated Encyclopedia*. London: Orbis, 1980.

Clifford, Terry. *Tibetan Buddhist Medicine and Psychiatry: The Diamond Healing*. York Beach, Me.: Samuel Weiser, 1984.

Franz, Marie-Louise von. *Number and Time*. Evanston, Ill.: Northwestern University Press, 1974.

———. *On Dreams und Death*. Boston and London: Shambhala, 1986.

Fremantle, Francesca, and Chögyam Trungpa. *The Tibetan Book of the Dead*. Boston and London: Shambhala, 1975.

Grey, Margot. *Return from Death: An Exploration of the Near-Death Experience*. London: Arkana, 1986.

Grof, Stanislav, and Christina Grof. *Beyond Death: The Gates of Consciousness*. E. P. Dutton: New York, 1980.

Grof, Stanislav, and Joan Halifax. *The Human Encounter with Death*. New York: E. P. Dutton, 1978.

Holck, Frederick H., ed. *Death and Eastern Thought: Understanding Death in Eastern Religions and Philosophies*. Nashville: Abingdon Press, 1974.

Houston, Jean. *The Possible Human*. Los Angeles: J. P. Tarcher, 1982.

Jung, C. G. *Memories, Dreams, Reflections*. Recorded and edited by Aniela Jaffé. Translated by Richard and Clara Winston. New York: Pantheon Books, 1961.

Kaplan, Amy. "The Hidden Dance." Master's thesis, Antioch University, Yellow Springs, Ohio, 1986.

Kübler-Ross, Elisabeth. *Questions and Answers on Death and Dying*. New York: Macmillan, 1974.

———. *Death, the Final Stage of Growth*. Englewood Cliffs, N.J.: Prentice Hall, 1975.

———. *On Death and Dying*. London: Tavistock Publications, 1976.

———. *To Live Until We Say Goodbye*. Englewood Cliffs, N.J.: Prentice-Hall, 1978.

———. *Living with Death and Dying*. New York: Macmillan, 1981.

Levine, Stephen. *Meetings at the Edge: Conversations with the Grieving and the Dying, the Healing and the Healed*. New York: Anchor Books, 1984.

———. *Who Dies: An Investigation of Conscious Living and Dying*. New York: Doubleday, 1982.

Little, Deborah W. *Home Care for the Dying*. New York: Doubleday, 1985.

Ludwig, A. "Altered States of Consciousness." In *Altered States of Consciousness*, edited by Charles Tart. New York: Wiley, 1969.

Mindell, Arnold. *Dreambody*. Santa Monica, Calif.: Sigo Press. 1982. London: Penguin Arkana, 1988.

———. *Working with the Dreaming Body*. London: Routledge & Kegan Paul, 1984. London and New York: Penguin Arkana, 1988.

———. *River's Way*. London: Routledge & Kegan Paul, 1985. London and New York: Penguin Arkana, 1988.

———. *The Dreambody in Relationships*. London: Routledge & Kegan Paul, 1987. London and New York: Penguin Arkana, 1988.

———. *City Shadows: Psychological Interventions in Psychiatry*. London: Routledge & Kegan Paul, 1988. London and New York: Penguin Arkana, 1988.

———. *The Year I: Global Process Work with Planetary Myths and Structures*. London and New York: Penguin Arkana, 1989.

———. *Working on Yourself Alone: Inner Dreambodywork*. London and New York: Penguin Arkana, 1989.

Monroe, Robert. *Journeys Out of the Body*. New York: Doubleday, 1977.

Moody, Raymond A. *Life After Life*. New York: Bantam Books, 1976.

Mullin, Glenn. *Death and Dying: The Tibetan Tradition*. London: Arkana, 1986.

Peat, David. *Synchronicity: The Bridge between Matter and Mind*. New York: Bantam Books, 1987.

Plum, Fred, and Jerome B. Posner. *The Diagnosis of Stupor and Coma*. 3d ed. Philadelphia: F. A. Davis, 1982.

Raheem, Aminah. "Process Oriented Acupressure." Unpublished manuscript. Zurich, May 1986.

Ring, Kenneth. *Heading toward Omega: In Search of the Meaning of the Near-Death Experience*. New York: Morrow, 1984.

Sabon, Michael, *Recollections of Death: A Medical Investigation*. New York: Harper & Row, 1982.

————. *The Near-Death Experience: A Medical Perspective*. New York: Lippincott, 1982.

Smith, Fritz. *Inner Bridges: Zero Balancing*. Atlanta: Humanics New Age, 1986.

Stein, Kathleen. "Last Rights." *Omni,* September 1987, p. 59.

Stoddard, Sandol. *The Hospice Movement*. New York: Vintage Books, 1978.

Tart, Charles. *Altered States of Consciousness*. New York: Wiley, 1969.

Tatelbaum, Judy. *The Courage to Grieve*. New York: Harper & Row, 1980.

Weinhold, Barry. *Altered States: An Explorer's Guide to Inner Space*. Denver: Love Publishing, 1987.

Zaleski, Carol. *Otherworld Journeys: Accounts of Near-Death Experience in Medieval and Modern Times*. New York: Oxford University Press, 1987.

Zenoff, Nancy. "The Mother's Experience After the Death of a Child." Ph.D. diss., Institute of Transpersonal Psychology, Menlo Park, Calif.

PENGUIN

ARKANA

NEW AGE BOOKS FOR MIND, BODY & SPIRIT

With over 200 titles currently in print, Arkana is the leading name in quality books for mind, body and spirit. Arkana encompasses the spirituality of both East and West, ancient and new. A vast range of interests is covered, including Psychology and Transformation, Health, Science and Mysticism, Women's Spirituality, Zen, Western Traditions and Astrology.

If you would like a catalogue of Arkana books, please write to:

Sales Dept. – Arkana
Penguin Books USA Inc.
375 Hudson Street
New York, NY 10014

Arkana Marketing Department
Penguin Books Ltd
27 Wrights Lane
London W8 5TZ

PENGUIN

ARKANA

NEW AGE BOOKS FOR MIND, BODY & SPIRIT

A SELECTION OF TITLES

The Revised Waite's Compendium of Natal Astrology
Alan Candlish

This completely revised edition retains the basic structure of Waite's classic work while making major improvements to accuracy and readability. With a new computer-generated Ephemeris, complete for the years 1900 to 2010, and a Table of Houses that now allows astrologers to choose between seven house systems, it provides all the information on houses, signs and planets the astrologer needs to draw up and interpret a full natal chart.

Aromatherapy for Everyone   Robert Tisserand

The therapeutic value of essential oils was recognized as far back as Ancient Egyptian times. Today there is an upsurge in the use of these fragrant and medicinal oils to soothe and heal both mind and body. Here is a comprehensive guide to every aspect of aromatherapy by the man whose name is synonymous with its practice and teaching.

Tao Te Ching   The Richard Wilhelm Edition

Encompassing philosophical speculation and mystical reflection, the *Tao Te Ching* has been translated more often than any other book except the Bible, and more analysed than any other Chinese classic. Richard Wilhelm's acclaimed 1910 translation is here made available in English.

The Book of the Dead   E. A. Wallis Budge

Intended to give the deceased immortality, the Ancient Egyptian *Book of the Dead* was a vital piece of 'luggage' on the soul's journey to the other world, providing for every need: victory over enemies, the procurement of friendship and – ultimately – entry into the kingdom of Osiris.

Yoga: Immortality and Freedom   Mircea Eliade

Eliade's excellent volume explores the tradition of yoga with exceptional directness and detail. 'One of the most important and exhaustive single-volume studies of the major ascetic techniques of India and their history yet to appear in English' – *San Francisco Chronicle*

PENGUIN

ARKANA

NEW AGE BOOKS FOR MIND, BODY & SPIRIT

A SELECTION OF TITLES

Weavers of Wisdom: Women Mystics of the Twentieth Century
Anne Bancroft

Throughout history women have sought answers to eternal questions about existence and beyond – yet most gurus, philosophers and religious leaders have been men. Through exploring the teachings of fifteen women mystics – each with her own approach to what she calls 'the truth that goes beyond the ordinary' – Anne Bancroft gives a rare, cohesive and fascinating insight into the diversity of female approaches to mysticism.

Dynamics of the Unconscious: Seminars in Psychological Astrology II
Liz Greene and Howard Sasportas

The authors of The *Development of the Personality* team up again to show how the dynamics of depth psychology interact with your birth chart. They shed new light on the psychology and astrology of aggression and depression – the darker elements of the adult personality that we must confront if we are to grow to find the wisdom within.

The Myth of the Eternal Return: Cosmos and History   Mircea Eliade

'A luminous, profound, and extremely stimulating work ... Eliade's thesis is that ancient man envisaged events not as constituting a linear, progressive history, but simply as so many creative repetitions of primordial archetypes ... This is an essay which everyone interested in the history of religion and in the mentality of ancient man will have to read. It is difficult to speak too highly of it' – Theodore H. Gaster in *Review of Religion*

The Second Krishnamurti Reader   Edited by Mary Lutyens

In this reader bringing together two of Krishnamurti's most popular works, *The Only Revolution* and *The Urgency of Change*, the spiritual teacher who rebelled against religion points to a new order arising when we have ceased to be envious and vicious. Krishnamurti says, simply: 'When you are not, love is.' 'Seeing,' he declares, 'is the greatest of all skills.' In these pages, gently, he helps us to open our hearts and eyes.

PENGUIN

ARKANA

NEW AGE BOOKS FOR MIND, BODY & SPIRIT

A SELECTION OF TITLES

A Course in Miracles
The Course, Workbook for Students and Manual for Teachers

Hailed as 'one of the most remarkable systems of spiritual truth available today', *A Course in Miracles* is a self-study course designed to shift our perceptions, heal our minds and change our behaviour, teaching us to experience miracles – 'natural expressions of love' – rather than problems generated by fear in our lives.

Fire in the Heart   Kyriacos C. Markides

A sequel to *The Magus of Strovolus* and *Homage to the Sun*, *Fire in the Heart* centres on Daskalos, the Cypriot healer and miracle-worker and his successor-designate Kostas. The author, who has witnessed much that is startling in his years with the two magi, believes humanity may today be on the verge of a revolution in consciousness 'more profound than the Renaissance and the Enlightenment combined.'

Arthur and the Sovereignty of Britain: Goddess and Tradition on the Mabinogion   Caitlín Matthews

Rich in legend and the primitive magic of the Celtic Otherworld, the stories of the *Mabinogion* heralded the first flowering of European literature and became the source of Arthurian legend. Caitlín Matthews illuminates these stories, shedding light on Sovereignty, the Goddess of the Land and the spiritual principle of the Feminine.

Shamanism: Archaic Techniques of Ecstasy   Mircea Eliade

Throughout Siberia and Central Asia, religious life traditionally centres around the figure of the shaman: magician and medicine man, healer and miracle-doer, priest and poet. 'Has become the standard work on the subject and justifies its claim to be the first book to study the phenomenon over a wide field and in a properly religious context' – *The Times Literary Supplement*

PENGUIN

ARKANA

NEW AGE BOOKS FOR MIND, BODY & SPIRIT

A SELECTION OF TITLES

Head Off Stress: Beyond the Bottom Line
D. E. Harding

Learning to head off stress takes no time at all and is impossible to forget – all it requires is that we dare take a fresh look at ourselves. This infallible and revolutionary guide from the author of *On Having No Head* – whose work C. S. Lewis described as 'highest genius' – shows how.

Shadows in the Cave Graham Dunstan Martin

We can all recognize our friends in a crowd, so why can't we describe in words what makes a particular face unique? The answer, says Graham Dunstan Martin, is that our minds are not just computers: drawing constantly on a fund of tacit knowledge, we always *know* more than we can ever say. Consciousness, in fact, is at the very heart of the universe, and – like the earth itself – we are all aspects of a single universal mind.

The Magus of Strovolos: The Extraordinary World of a Spiritual Healer Kyriacos C. Markides

This vivid account introduces us to the rich and intricate world of Daskalos, the Magus of Strovolos – a true healer who draws upon a seemingly limitless mixture of esoteric teachings, psychology, reincarnation, demonology, cosmology and mysticism, from both East and West. 'This is a really marvellous book … one of the most extraordinary accounts of a "magical" personality since Ouspensky's account of Gurdjieff' – Colin Wilson

Meetings With Remarkable Men G. I. Gurdjieff

All that we know of the early life of Gurdjieff – one of the great spiritual masters of this century – is contained within these colourful and profound tales of adventure. The men who influenced his formative years had no claim to fame in the conventional sense; what made them remarkable was the consuming desire they all shared to understand the deepest mysteries of life.

PENGUIN

ARKANA

NEW AGE BOOKS FOR MIND, BODY & SPIRIT

A SELECTION OF TITLES

Working on Yourself Alone: Inner Dreambody Work
Arnold Mindell

Western psychotherapy and Eastern meditation are two contrasting ways of learning more about one's self. The first depends heavily on the powers of the therapist. *Process-oriented* meditation, however, can be used by the individual as a means of resolving conflicts and increasing awareness from within. Using meditation, dream work and yoga, this remarkable book offers techniques that you can develop on your own, allowing the growth of an individual method.

Neo-Astrology Michel Gauquelin

Michel Gauquelin's Neo-Astrology is a frugal science that discards much of the traditional horoscope, and suggests that five planets only – Saturn, Jupiter, Mars, Venus and the Moon – affect us. This important work shows that the French psychologist and statistician may be pointing towards nothing less than a new model of the universe.

Homage to the Sun: The Wisdom of the Magus of Strovolos
Kyriacos C. Markides

Homage to the Sun continues the adventure into the mysterious and extraordinary world of the spiritual teacher and healer Daskalos, the 'Magus of Strovolos'. The logical foundations of Daskalos' world of other dimensions are revealed to us – invisible masters, past-life memories and guardian angels, all explained by the Magus with great lucidity and scientific precision.

The Eagle's Gift Carlos Castaneda

In the sixth book in his astounding journey into sorcery, Castaneda returns to Mexico. Entering once more a world of unknown terrors, hallucinatory visions and dazzling insights, he discovers that he is to replace the Yaqui Indian don Juan as leader of the apprentice sorcerers – and learns of the significance of the Eagle.

PENGUIN

ARKANA

NEW AGE BOOKS FOR MIND, BODY & SPIRIT

A SELECTION OF TITLES

The Dreambody in Relationships Arnold Mindell

All of us communicate on several levels at once, and Mindell shows how much of our silent language conflicts with overt behaviour. He argues that bringing all the hidden parts of ourselves to awareness as they affect us is important for the well-being not only of our relationships but also of the community – indeed, the world – in which we live.

The Sacred Yew Anand Chetan and Diana Brueton

Recently it has been discovered that the yew can live for many thousands of years. *The Sacred Yew* is the inspiring story of one man's crusade to preserve this revered yet threatened tree and explain its importance to all our lives.

Be As You Are Sri Ramana Maharshi

'The ultimate truth is so simple.' This is the message of Sri Ramana Maharshi, one of India's most revered spiritual masters whose teachings, forty years after his death, are speaking to growing audiences worldwide. 'That sense of presence, of the direct communication of the truth so far as it can be put into words, is there on every page' – *Parabola*

In Search of the Miraculous: Fragments of an Unknown Teaching P. D. Ouspensky

Ouspensky's renowned, vivid and characteristically honest account of his work with Gurdjieff from 1915 to 1918. 'Undoubtedly a *tour de force*. To put entirely new and very complex cosmology and psychology into fewer than 400 pages, and to do this with a simplicity and vividness that makes the book accessible to any educated reader, is in itself something of an achievement' – *The Times Literary Supplement*